BEING WELL

foundations of lifelong
health & happiness

DR. DAWNA ARA

Copyright © 2024 Dawna Ara, LLC. All rights reserved

The information provided in this book is the opinion of the author and is for general purposes only. The information in this book does not replace medical, health, nutritional, or other competent professional advice and should not be used as a basis for making decisions about your health or the health of others. The reader should consult their medical doctor before adopting any of the suggestions in this book. No doctor-patient relationship is being established by your use of this book.

While the author and publisher have made every attempt to ensure the information in this book is correct and obtained from reliable resources at the time of publishing, the author and publisher are not responsible for any errors of omission, or for the results obtained from the use of this information.

No part of this book may be reproduced, or stored in a retrieval system, or transmitted in any form or by any means, electronic, mechanical, photocopying, recording, or otherwise, without express written permission of the publisher.

Cover design by: Dawna Ara

Printed in the United States of America

*To my parents who gave me wings,
and my kids, who anchored them.*

Contents

Intro 1
    My story 5
Rewire 9
    Brain basics 11
    Stuck on repeat 13
    Get comfortable with being uncomfortable 14
    Spot the scripts 15
    Put the scripts on trial 16
    Draft a new story 17
    Looking back 18
    Imagine it 18
    Reinvent yourself 21
    Focus on the good 23
    Unclutter your mind 26
    Additional resources 31
Eat 33
    Nutrients 34
    Principles of healthy eating 36
    Avoid ultra-processed food 38
    Eat minimally processed foods 40
    Eat real food 41
    Eat primarily plants 42
    Be vegicurious 43
    Ignore fat-free propaganda 44
    Eat healthy fats 46
    Avoid unhealthy fats 47
    Know the smoking points 49
    Eat the rainbow 51
    Drink more water 53

Be mindful of portion sizes 56
Eat at regular times 58
Shrink your eating window 59
Choose healthier cooking methods 60
Avoid pesticides 63
Buy antibiotic & hormone free meats 64
Prep your meals 66
Don't overcomplicate it 70
Enjoy your food 70

Move 73

Where to start 75
How much do you need? 76
What's the best kind of exercise? 76
Walking 79
Jogging / Running 80
Cycling 81
Swimming 82
Resistance bands 82
Yoga 83
Racket sports 84
Overcome exercise anxiety 85

Sleep 87

Sleep-wake cycle 89
Stages of sleep 90
How to sleep better 91
Get early morning sunlight 92
Limit caffeine intake 93
Avoid alcohol 95
Time your meals & eat for sleep 96
Move your body 99
Create sleep rituals 100
Bliss out your bedroom 102

v

Cool it down 104
Mind your screen time..106
Get it off your chest...107
Sync your slumber..108
Get out of bed 109
Meditate 111
Make love 113
Don't snack on sleep..115
Restful remedies 116

Relax **119**

The modern caveman's dilemma.................................120
Get familiar with your triggers....................................122
Know your symptoms 123
Burn off stress 124
Relax harder 125
Nourish your nerves 128
Choose healthier vices...131
Go play 132
Get your Zzzzzs...133
Lean on friends..133
Unplug 134
Master your time 135
Kindly decline 136

Detox..**139**

Detox 101 142
Signs you could use detox support..............................144
Stop putting toxins in your body 144
Flush out your body...145
Eat detox friendly foods 146
Eat lots of fiber 150
Eat organic whenever possible 151
Give your gut a break 152

vi

Boost with supplements 153
  Cut out liver-harming substances 158
  Exercise to support detoxification 161
  Prioritize sleep 162
  Find ways to unwind 163
  Dry brush your skin 164
  Get a massage 166
  Sit in a sauna 166
  Take an epsom salt bath 168
  Use an air purifier 169
  Invest in a water filter 170

Connect 173
  A brief history of communities 174
  Start with yourself 175
  Nurture your relationships 178
  Notice what you like 180
  Make new connections 182
  Pick your battles 183
  Rethink your top 5 184
  Be the influencer 185
  Pull the weeds 187
  Stay in touch 188

Pursue 191
  Why find your Ikigai? 192
  What do you love to do? 193
  What does the world need? 195
  What are you good at? 196
  What can you get paid for? 197
  Take action 198
  Find a mentor 201
  Follow your curiosity 202

Integrate 205

Rewire	206
Eat	206
Move	208
Sleep	209
Relax	210
Detox	211
Connect	213
Pursue	214
Final thoughts	214
Resources	**217**
References	**219**
About the author	**243**
What clients are saying	**245**

Health and happiness are natural consequences of self-love.

Intro

*Happiness is not something ready made.
It comes from your own actions.*

~ The Dalai Lama

What would you say if I asked you if you wanted to live a long and healthy life? Would you say yes? Most of us want nothing more than lifelong health and happiness for ourselves and loved ones. For me, the idea of living out my golden years on a sunny beach with robust health is alluring. But for some, the trajectory of life is muddied by chronic disease. Fatigue, stress, anxiety, depression, pain, digestive and hormonal problems, and extra weight are the American norm. Why? Because, as a society, we're overworked and sleep deprived, overfed on highly processed foods and under-exercised. Lack of deep connection with others and the denial of our higher purpose dampens our quality of life. Does it have to be this way? Absolutely not, and this book will teach you how to be the exception.

BEING WELL

I wrote this book as a response to an alarming trend I've observed over 15 years of working with patients—modern life is the blueprint for disease. Wake up, rush out the door, eat unhealthy food, return home late at night exhausted, have a drink to relax, watch TV, then head to bed only to repeat it all the next day. Living this way for a short time may not affect your health, but overtime, chronic disease develops, and it becomes harder to bounce back. The issue isn't that you lack the ability to change—it's that you're stuck on autopilot and unhealthy habits are incredibly challenging to break.

While genetics play a role, it is your lifestyle that inevitably directs your health.[1] The choices you make either bring you closer to optimal health or drive you down the road to illness. Don't believe me? Even the Center for Disease Control and Prevention (CDC) acknowledges several diseases and symptoms are directly linked to lifestyle.[2] The top 10 lifestyle related diseases are as follows;

- **Heart disease:** unhealthy eating, lack of exercise, and smoking
- **Stroke:** poor diet, sedentary lifestyle.
- **Type 2 Diabetes:** obesity, poor diet, lack of exercise.
- **Obesity:** overeating, poor diet, lack of exercise, stress.
- **Hypertension (High blood pressure):** poor diet, high salt, obesity, stress.
- **Chronic Obstructive Pulmonary Disease (COPD):** smoking, long-term exposure to pollutants.

INTRO

- **Cancer (lung, colorectal, breast):** smoking, diet, sedentary lifestyle.
- **Osteoporosis:** poor diet (low intake of calcium), lack of weight-bearing exercise, smoking.
- **Fatty Liver:** obesity, high intake of alcohol, high intake of refined vegetable oils, high-sugar diet.
- **Depression:** lack of exercise, poor diet, chronic stress.

Scared? Don't be. You're not doomed to suffer from any of the above conditions. Many diseases are preventable and possibly even reversible. The secret to good health is learning techniques and then diligently applying them to your life. Like learning to ride a bike or type on the computer, health and happiness are skills anyone can master. They take constant practice and the ability to make good decisions repeatedly.

This book aims to help you do just that—design your life so that good health and happiness are the direct results of your habits. In other words, true well-being becomes the default state of your lifestyle. You won't have to move to the Himalayas and become a monk; once you learn the process, you can easily integrate these practices into your daily life and notice profound benefits.

There's a lot of information out there making health complicated; take three boxes of supplements, don't take any supplements; eat a carnivore diet, eat a vegan diet, eat kale, don't eat kale, do a three day water fast, calculate your VO2 max, sit in a bath filled with ice water every day. While these things can be beneficial, they're intimidating and misleading to the person trying to figure out where to start. You did not get sick, gain weight, become fatigued, anxious, depressed or whatever is ailing you because you weren't taking a daily ice bath. You got sick due to smaller, yet more powerful daily habits. If you're constantly eating junk food, watching screens for hours, and rarely exercising, then sitting in an ice bath isn't going to solve your health problems.

Building health is much like building a house. You have to start with a foundation before you put up a frame. Even if you put up walls made out of the strongest materials, the house will eventually collapse if it doesn't have a strong foundation.

So then where do you start? Start with the basics—your mind, body, and spirit. These are your starting points, providing a solid foundation for building health. We're not treating disease—*we are creating a baseline of health so your body is more resistant to disease.*

As you make your way through this book, you'll find yourself more resilient to stress and less reactive to your thoughts and emotions. You'll find nutrition to be less confusing and movement to be fun and nearly effortless. These foundations will help you cultivate a deep connection with yourself and your loved ones to live a richer and more meaningful life.

This book is filled with simple concepts and ideas that you can practice overtime instead of trying to make dramatic changes overnight. Over time, as you become comfortable with the foundations, you can incorporate advanced practices like ice bathing to continue improving your health.

INTRO

MY STORY

I know all about slipping into unhealthy routines and habits. Not too long ago, I was overworked, going back to school to get my doctorate, pregnant with my second child, and sandwiched between raising littles and taking care of aging parents. I still ate relatively healthy and exercised but wasn't sleeping well and had little time for friends and family. The stress was real, but I was addicted to the adrenaline rush, and frankly, I wasn't feeling bad enough to change my patterns.

The stress amplified, and once my second son was born I could barely get out of bed. A plague of anxiety and exhaustion took over my body. I remember waking up in a pool of sweat and a deep rhythmic kick in my chest, like a ticking time bomb that rattled my entire body. For the first time in my life, I thought I would die. After a long list of medical tests, it turned out I had postpartum thyroiditis, an autoimmune disease in which the immune system mistakenly attacks the thyroid gland. Postpartum thyroiditis presents with a racing, pounding heart, anxiety, extreme fatigue, and hot flashes.

I knew autoimmune disease well. It was something I treated in my clinic daily. I knew my lifestyle and the stress of having a baby and being postpartum were significant triggers. More importantly, I knew I could reverse it by changing my life.

I immediately began caring for myself, utilizing the foundations laid out in this book. I changed my mindset, started eating better and moving more, slept as much as possible, managed stress by asking for help, reconnected with loved ones, and found myself again by doing things I love. My health quickly turned around. Once I started to feel better, I examined how I got there in the first place—my health crumbled because I didn't build a strong enough foundation. On top of that, I kept pushing myself without recharging until my batteries ultimately died.

Looking back, getting sick was a blessing. It allowed me to rebuild my health in a way that made me stronger and more energetic. Every part of my being benefited from building a solid foundation in overall well-being. And now that I have experienced this as a patient, I am humbled and empathetic to what I now know is needless suffering. The principles in this book are simple yet can prevent you or anyone from hitting rock bottom like I did. If I can overcome my unhealthy habits, so can you.

So let's start building your foundation!

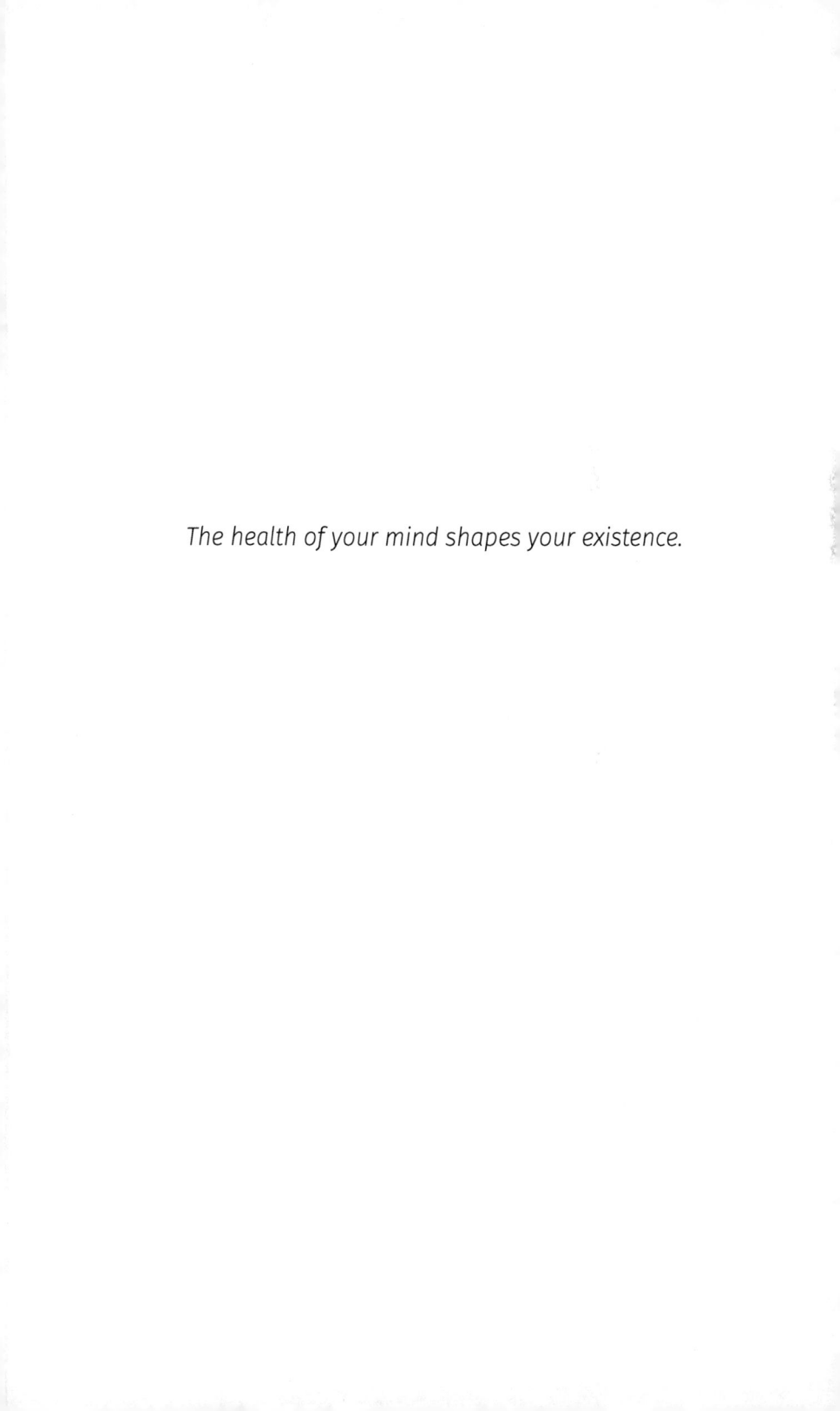

The health of your mind shapes your existence.

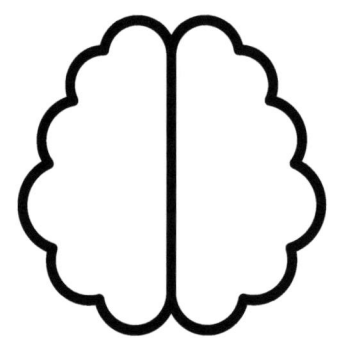

Rewire

Believe you can, and you're halfway there.
~ Theodore Roosevelt

Want to improve your well-being? Then start with your mind. The world's healthiest individuals use techniques like visualization, prayer, and meditation to shape their futures. Physical health, emotional resilience, and overall happiness all spring from the health of your mind.

Your mind is the foundation of who you are. It's the birthplace of your personality and where your beliefs, thoughts, emotions, behaviors, attitudes, and habits reside. It guides every decision you make, every goal you chase, and every challenge you face.

If you want to change your life in any way, start with your mind.

Want to lose weight? Use your mind to change your habits. Habits are born through repetition and nurtured in the mind. Health conscious individuals developed habits that naturally guide them towards healthy choices. They don't struggle to eat healthy, go to bed early, or exercise because they've trained their minds to crave these things automatically.

Would you like to be one of these people who's healthy habits are on autopilot, requiring little effort or conscious thought?

If unhealthy habits are holding you back, wouldn't you change them so you could live a better life? Imagine waking up without an alarm clock, energetic, pain free, and looking forward to your day. Imagine growing old and thriving well into your 80s, 90s, and above with little to no disease. With a little work up front, you can make this your reality.

To change your habits you have to understand what influences them. Why do you snack late at night? Why do you stay up late when you know you have to wake up early? Why do you constantly argue with your partner? Habits are heavily influenced by thoughts, and behind every thought is a belief you may not even be aware of.

Beliefs are stories you tell yourself about the world. They're based on observations and assumptions, not hard facts. In other words, you don't view the world as it is; you view it through a lens morphed by yours or other people's experiences.

Where do these stories come from? They come from the voices of your caregivers, siblings, friends, spouses, teachers, leaders, bosses, and coworkers. They come from the shows you watch, the music you listen to, the experiences you've had, and the choices you've made.

You have beliefs about many things, but we'll focus on the ones you have about yourself. These narratives are the most critical determinants of your life's success. They shape your perception of your abilities, setting the boundaries of what you believe is attainable. Said another way, you can not change a habit, or achieve something you want unless you believe it's possible.

Beliefs however, are not set in stone; they're open to change and evolution. So even if you don't believe you can improve your life now, you can change that belief by challenging or disproving the evidence that initially shaped your belief.[1] If you want to change your habits around health and happiness, you must dissect, understand, and, if necessary, rewrite those deeply seated beliefs to become the person you want to be. But first, let's go over some basics so you understand how beliefs and habits can be changed.

BRAIN BASICS

The brain we develop reflects the life we lead.
~ The Dalai Lama

Your brain is a network of billions of tiny cells working together to transmit information. These cells are called neurons and chat with each other by sending messages across gaps called synapses. Neurons like to send messages at the same time as other neurons. Paired neurons get really good at communicating with each other and become glued together. The more they communicate, the stronger their glue becomes.

When you try to change a belief or habit, you soften the glue that holds neurons together. You weaken the bond so they eventually get disconnected and in turn, break a habit or belief. Long-held beliefs are harder to pull apart because they've been glued together for years. However, it can be done with deliberate and consistent repetition. If you want to change a belief, you must tell yourself a story that contradicts the old belief and rehearse it over and over and over until you really believe it. Introducing new perspectives and reflecting on them encourages neurons to uncouple, and different ones to pair up and form new bonds.

The brain can also form new neurons in a process called neurogenesis.[2] 'Neuro' means neuron, and 'genesis' means birth. Many things can support neurogenesis, such as exercise, diet, stress, age, genetics, and engaging in activities that challenge existing beliefs. So by challenging your belief, you're forming new brain cells.

The process of rewiring your brain is hard work. You can't change your habits by dabbling in a few activities here and there, you have to continue doing them long enough to cross a threshold. Changing beliefs takes time, repetition, and effort, and most people give up on themselves far too early.

REWIRE

STUCK ON REPEAT

I think I can, I think I can, I think I can.
~ The Little Engine That Could

Beliefs, along with thoughts, ideas, and assumptions are patterns of thinking that we call mindsets.[3] You can think of mindsets like the default setting your mind returns to when life gets glitchy. Mindsets are like radio stations that play the same songs over and over again in your head. But these songs aren't just background noise—they're the influential soundtracks of your life. They drive your behaviors and actions. While there's thousands of radio stations playing all kinds of songs, your mind is tuned to only one, filtering how you see the world. Imagine if you only heard country music, or rap, or jazz; your entire view of music would be based off that one genre.

Like songs, mindsets can direct your mood and outlook. Some are inspiring, encouraging you to follow your dreams, while others tell another story, based off fear and doubt. When a negative song gets stuck on repeat, it becomes a barrier, blocking you from seeing what's truly attainable.

Think back to a time you faced something difficult. Maybe it concerned work, family, health, or a relationship. What song was playing in your head at that time? Were you determined to tackle the difficulty with dedication and hard work, or did you retreat, believing you didn't have the skills to make it happen?

If you doubt your ability to succeed at something, you're less likely to try, thereby validating your belief. However, even if a tiny part of you envisions success, you're more likely to persist and find creative ways to make things happen.

The good news is that you're not stuck with your current mindset. You can change the station. So even if the only song currently playing is "I'm Not Good Enough," you can shut it off by recognizing it, questioning why it's playing, and then rewriting it to influence your life in better ways.

GET COMFORTABLE WITH BEING UNCOMFORTABLE

Most everything that you want is just outside your comfort zone.
~ Jack Canfield

The process of change is inherently uncomfortable. Many struggle to change because they don't want to experience discomfort. However, the discomfort is only temporarily until what you are trying to change becomes a habit. To understand what I'm saying, try this simple exercise;

- Grab a pen and a piece of paper and write down your name.

- Now switch, and write your name with your non-dominant hand. For most of us, writing with our non-dominant hand feels awkward.

- Put it back in your dominant hand and again write down your name. I bet this feels more natural, and your writing is more legible.

Yet, this is why so many people fail to make real change—we'd rather return to what's comfortable and easy. However, what you practice you become. If you wanted to get good at writing with your non-dominant hand, you would have to push through the discomfort and continue writing with it. At some point your writing would improve.

The same is true when trying to change your habits around health. If you want to lose weight and keep it off, you need a consistent daily practice of healthy habits. You can't expect the weight to melt off after one day of exercise and healthy eating. It requires stepping out of your comfort zone and diligently practicing healthy habits day after day, month after month until they become second nature. Time and repetition is not only how you change your body, but it's how you rewire your brain to love your new, healthy habits.

Below are ways to rewire your mind and change the beliefs that are holding you back from transforming your health.

SPOT THE SCRIPTS

The first step in changing limiting mindsets is spotting the scripts that are playing over and over in your head. Listen for statements you say to yourself such as "I can't" or "I'm not" or I'll never." These scripts stem from stories that don't entirely reflect objective reality. They're filtered through our interpretations, expectations, frameworks, and simplifications of reality. Ask yourself the following questions;

- What beliefs do you have about yourself that may be holding you back from achieving health and happiness?
- Do you notice any recurring negative thoughts or self-talk patterns?
- How do these beliefs impact your actions, choices, and goals?
- Are there specific areas of your life where you encounter these limiting beliefs?
- How long have you held onto these beliefs, and where did they come from?

PUT THE SCRIPTS ON TRIAL

Cross examine the script and you'll likely find very little evidence for it. Whatever you do find is likely outdated and needs to be reassessed. Examine the data like a scientist.

- What's really true in the situation?
- What isn't true?
- What evidence do you have that supports these limiting beliefs?

REWIRE

- Have any experiences or past events reinforced these beliefs?
- Can you find any counterexamples or contradictory evidence challenging these beliefs?
- How realistic and accurate are these beliefs when objectively observed?
- What alternative perspectives or interpretations could be considered?

DRAFT A NEW STORY

Once you've spotted and examined the script, write yourself a new story. Replace "I can't" and "I'm not" with "I can" and "I am."

- What new, empowering beliefs would you like to adopt in place of the limiting beliefs?
- How do these new beliefs align with your values, aspirations, and goals?
- What evidence supports these empowering beliefs?
- How can you challenge and question limiting beliefs when they arise?
- What strategies or techniques can you use to reframe and replace negative self-talk with positive affirmations?

BEING WELL

LOOKING BACK

Looking over your responses, what insights or realizations have you gained about your limiting beliefs?

- What are the potential consequences of holding onto these limiting beliefs?

- What positive outcomes can you envision by challenging and replacing these beliefs?

- Set one or two actionable goals to challenge your limiting beliefs and foster new empowering beliefs. Keep them specific, measurable, achievable, relevant, and time-bound (SMART goals).

Remember that changing mindsets is a gradual process, requiring time, self-awareness, reflection, practice, and consistent effort. By consciously examining and challenging your mindset, you can reshape it to align with your goals and values around health.

IMAGINE IT

Don't just think outside of the box.
Visualize a world without boxes.
~ Unknown

One of the most powerful tools you can use to change your habits is mental imagery.[4] Mental imagery, like visualization, is the art of daydreaming. It's where your imagination runs free to create vivid movies in your mind. It may not seem like you're doing much, but you're actually rewiring your brain every time you do it to get what you want.[5]

When I first tell people about the power of mental imagery, I usually get some resistance. "You mean I can just close my eyes and imagine myself better?" Yes, that's exactly what I'm saying. Mental imagery is a form of rehearsal that primes your brain for better or for worse. This means if you're constantly visualizing negative outcomes, then they'll likely come true as well.[6]

How does it work? Several studies have shown that the area of the brain responsible for imagination is the same area that deals with real-life experience.[7] In other words, the mind doesn't know the difference between real and imagined.

Have you ever woken up from a bad dream sweating, breathing hard, with a racing heart? That was your mind creating reality. Your body physically changes in response to your dreams. The same scenario plays out with your thoughts. If you visualize yourself healthy, your brain and body will act in ways that match that imagery.[8]

However, you can't just imagine yourself a millionaire then sit on the couch and wait for it to happen. You still have to take action and work towards your goal. But visualizing will change areas in your brain that help you stay on track to achieving that goal.

Why not visualize a healthier version of yourself so your mind can align with that vision and turn it into reality?

In crafting your health vision, be as specific as possible and visualize every detail of every element you want. Don't just see something; attach emotions, sensations, smells, and sounds for stronger connections. Make it vivid and real. Studies show the more you feel, the more chemical changes occur in your body.[9] If you have trouble visualizing what you want, use pictures. Maybe you have old photos of yourself that you wish to return to or images of someone you inspire to be like. You can do this in your journal or make a vision board with pictures and visuals to look at daily. Here's how to do it;

- Describe what you want. Be detailed and thorough.

- Now imagine it already happening. What do you look like? Where are you? What do you see around you? What sounds do you hear? What do you feel? What do you taste? What do you smell? Who is with you?

- Make it emotional with feelings of joy, satisfaction, pride, happiness, etc. Really feel these emotions in your body.

- How would having what you want benefit your life? What could you do that you can't do now? Take time to think about it and write down everything you come up with.

Practice mental imagery every day—when you wake up and before going to bed. Read through your visualization list, pause and really imagine yourself the way you want to be. Soon you'll start to believe it and align your life with your vision.

REWIRE

REINVENT YOURSELF

The only person you are destined to become is the person you decide to be.

~ Ralph Waldo Emerson

Not long ago, a woman named Emily walked into my office with back pain, fatigue, trouble sleeping, and weight gain. The initial assessment revealed some pretty self-defeating habits. Among them was Emily's nightly glass of wine, which she claimed helped her relax and fall asleep.

However, the very wine she leaned on was linked to all her ailments. I asked her if she could let it go, and without a pause, she said, "Absolutely not." It was one of the only things she looked forward to, and she couldn't imagine her life without it.

Emily was having an identity crisis. She didn't want to give up her nightly wine because she identified as a wine drinker. On top of that, she didn't see wine as a problem; she saw it as the solution to her problems.

I asked her what was more important; drinking the wine or getting rid of her symptoms. She thought about it briefly, then said "getting rid of the symptoms," but was sincerely scared of what life would be like without wine.

Our actions are largely dictated by how we perceive ourselves.[10] Health-conscious individuals are more likely to exercise, eat healthy, and get regular checkups. A devout Christian likely attends church, prays, and reads the bible.

BEING WELL

To help Emily shift her mindset, I proposed an exercise in self-perception. What if, instead of identifying as a wine drinker, Emily saw herself as health-conscious, a person who prioritizes well-being above anything else? To make the transition more comfortable, she could drink non-alcoholic beverages from her wine glass, allowing her to maintain the ritual without consequence. Emily agreed to give it a shot.

By changing her self-perception, Emily's actions began to align with her new identity. From that change came her desired outcome—better sleep, more energy, reduced back pain, and weight loss. But the transformation wasn't just physical. As she redefined who she was and what she valued, Emily set off a domino effect—knocking down other habits that no longer aligned with her new identity. Her entire life transformed because of a simple shift in perspective.

Below is an exercise to help you transform your health by reinventing your self-image. Answer the following questions;

- What habits or behaviors are affecting your well-being?
- What benefits or relief do they provide?
- What negative outcomes or health issues are connected to this habit?
- How do you currently identify in relation to this habit?
- Can you envision an identity shift that would promote a healthier lifestyle?
- Write down what is more important to you: Continuing the habit or improving your well-being. Why?

- Describe any concerns or fears you have about letting go of this habit.

- Think of individuals who embody the identity you aspire to be like. What habits and behaviors do they exhibit?

- What are some ways you can transition out of the habit while preserving parts of the ritual you enjoy?

FOCUS ON THE GOOD

*For every minute you are angry
you lose sixty seconds of happiness.*

~ Ralph Waldo Emerson

The human brain is inherently wired to focus on the negative. This mechanism is called the negativity bias, and is thought to have helped our ancestors recognize and prioritize danger.[11] However, our lives are far safer today than they were thousands of years ago. We're not getting chased by massive predators nor hunting in atrocious weather so we don't need to be primed to respond to so much danger.

But evolution is slow and hasn't caught up with modern living. Being wired to focus on negativism can lead to stress, anxiety, and pessimistic beliefs about your own abilities.[12] Actively seeking things to appreciate can counteract our innate tendency towards pessimism.[13] It shifts your attention from minor details to a broader, more optimistic view of life.

BEING WELL

While focusing on the good doesn't invalidate the genuine pain and difficulties we face, it can change your outlook, reframe a bad experience, and help you find comfort even in life's most challenging moments.

Having a positive outlook is associated with a lower incidence of stress and anxiety, reduced inflammation, lower blood pressure and glucose levels, higher pain tolerance, increased resilience to trauma, higher self-esteem, motivation, a better immune system, better sleep, and increased longevity.[14, 15, 16, 17]

Let me tell you about William, a construction worker not really into self-improvement, but came to see me out of desperation. His neck and shoulders reflected his current state of being—weighed down by the burdens of life. A series of unfortunate events left him jaded and unable to see the good in his life. Talking to him was like pulling teeth.

He didn't come to me for a lecture on well-being, but luckily, he would do anything to get out of physical pain, including the new-age stuff I was about to suggest.

I told him that sometimes, a shift in perspective can trigger the release of both physical and emotional pain. I suggested he actively look for things to love and appreciate, such as the friends in his life, the clothes on his back, or the food on his plate. While focusing on the positive wouldn't solve his problems, it could help release the negative emotions attached to them. Both pessimism and optimism are states of mind. He could either choose to see the good in his life or not.

William rolled his eyes but I could see the wheels spinning behind them. I knew he knew there was something to what I was saying. He just needed some time to process it. William gave in to my requests, and the next time I saw him the tightness in his neck and shoulders had softened, as did his outlook on life.

When you consistently engage in practices such as gratitude, love, or appreciation, areas in your brain associated with positive emotions, memory, and overall well-being grow stronger.[18] In contrast, those associated with stress, conflict, and anxiety begin to dissolve. William's brain changed in response to his new habits, as can yours. Below are effective methods to train your brain to focus more on the good and less on the bad.

- **Keep a Journal:** Take a couple of minutes each day to reflect on the positive aspects of your day. What went well? Next, write down a few things, no matter how big or small, that you're grateful for. It could be a kind gesture from a stranger, a meal you savored, a call from a loved one, or a warm blanket, etc. You can write in your journal any time of the day, but doing it right before bed can help you have a better night's sleep.

- **Let People Know You Appreciate Them:** Find things you like about the people you interact with and give them a complement. Even if you can only think of their haircut, let them know. This helps prime your brain to spot what you like about people rather than what you don't. It not only strengthens the bond between you and your loved ones, but it can significantly improve your overall health.

- **Make a Gratitude Bowl:** Put a small bowl out somewhere visible in your home. Every day, write down one thing you're grateful for or appreciate on a small piece of paper. Put the paper in the bowl, and over time, watch the bowl grow with reasons to be thankful. You can read through them at the end of a week, month, or year as a reminder of all the good things in your life.

- **Visual Reminders:** Decorate your house with meaningful photographs and objects that bring you joy and make you smile. The brain associates visual cues with emotions. Constantly seeing things you love creates a habit loop that reinforces positive feelings, happiness, and gratitude whenever you look at them.

UNCLUTTER YOUR MIND

*The thing about meditation is:
You become more and more you.*

~ David Lynch

Have you ever been so entrenched in thought that paying attention to the world around you seems nearly impossible? Or has your busy mind robbed you of sleep, replaying embarrassing memories or preparing you for everything that could go wrong the next day?

If this sounds familiar, meditation might be the solution for you. Try this: close your eyes, sit still for a minute, and see what comes up. You probably noticed a bunch of random thoughts. That's typical, but there's a mute button, and I can show you how to find it.

Meditation is a refocusing practice that has its roots in Buddhism. It's a powerful tool that brings your attention back from the past or future and trains it to focus on the moment. We tend to make a bigger deal out of it than it is, which is why so many of us struggle when we're first learning to meditate.

The difficulty of meditation lies in its simplicity—sit still and pause the stories in your head. It's torture for those of us with rushing minds, but the payoff is priceless—inner peace and a calmer state of being.

The good news is that you don't need to spend hours meditating under a Bodhi tree to see benefits. Even as little as five minutes a day can decrease stress, depression, worry, and anxiety as well as improve heart rate variability, enhance attention, improve memory, and your overall mood.[19, 20, 21]

I admit I wasn't the biggest fan of meditation when I first started. Back then, my mind was like a cluttered bedroom, with thoughts and worries piled high from corner to corner. My sister suggested I learn to meditate, but I resisted. Who has time to chant ohm while the world flies by in the fast lane? But, when the mental chatter dominated every waking hour, I caved and listened to a guided meditation for anxiety. My brain ran a thousand miles per minute. I tried to focus on my breath, but an imaginary story about the future kept stealing my attention. I hated meditation. I was frustrated and it was all my sister's fault.

But near the end of the meditation, the teacher offered a profound insight. She said distractions are your gift. Instead of being frustrated by their presence, be thankful. Without them, you wouldn't be able to practice meditation. Losing focus and refocusing is the very process that rewires your brain. The more you do it, the longer the pause between thoughts will become, and the better you'll get.

A lightbulb went on in my head. Meditation isn't about making all thoughts stop. It's about realizing you're having a thought, letting it go, and returning to the present moment when you get distracted by it. That's all. I didn't need to sit there with an empty head for 20 long minutes. Once I realized I was lost in thought, I could pause, return to my breath, and replace the distracting thought with a better one.

The teacher's words released some of the anxiety and frustration I was feeling around meditating and allowed me to relax for the remainder of the session.

Soon, I was meditating twice a day when I woke up and went to bed. Surprisingly, I looked forward to those 10-minute sessions where I could pause and work on my mind. And that teacher was right; the more I meditated, the better I got. Not so much at meditation; I still get distracted every session. But what I did get better at was life.

Meditation taught me how to clean up and organize my mental room. It freed my mind so I could prioritize thoughts that made me a better, happier person. Here's a quick introductory meditation you can do anywhere to calm your mind;

- Find a quiet space where you can sit comfortably or lay down for the next five minutes without distractions.

- Close your eyes and take a deep breath in from your nose for a count of four, hold it for a count of seven, then exhale slowly for the count of eight through the mouth. Repeat this two more times.

- Bring your awareness to your body starting from your head and moving downwards.

- Feel the sensations as you scan down your body. Notice areas of tension and imagine them releasing and letting go.

- When you are finished with the body scan bring your attention back to your breath for one full minute. Don't try to change how you are breathing, just observe.

- Notice the air flow in and out of your nose and the rise and fall of your chest. When your mind starts to wander, just bring it back to your breath.

- Next, spend a moment focusing on all the things you're grateful for. It could be as simple as the sun shinning on your face or as significant as a loved one. Feel the gratitude fill your body and expand outwards. Let the gratitude feel the entire room, then your entire town, country, earth, and feel it expand out into the universe.

BEING WELL

- When you're finished, slowly start to bring your attention back to the present moment.
- Take a few more deep breaths as you wiggle your fingers and toes.
- Open your eyes. You should feel a sense of calmness and peace within yourself.

ADDITIONAL RESOURCES

Scan the QR code below to access free guided meditations, worksheets, and additional resources for each section of this book.

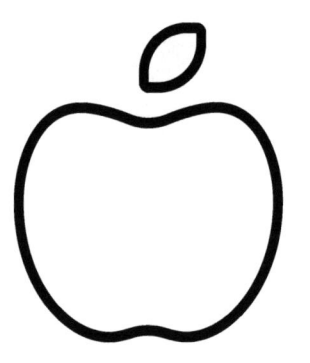

Eat

Tell me what you eat, and I will tell you what you are.

~ Jean Anthelme Brillat-Savarin

In all my years of practice, I am still amazed by how many people don't think food has anything to do with their health. Food is literally the thing you put into your body three or so times a day. Every single cell in your body is made from the food you eat. If you eat inflammatory foods daily for months, years, or even decades, you're going to develop a chronic disease. On the other hand, if you've been feeding your body nourishing food and staying hydrated, chances are your diet isn't causing ill health and is likely preventing it.

    The word 'diet' can be triggering and carries a lot of emotional weight. It's much bigger than what you see on a nutrition label—calories, protein, carbs, and fat. Your diet is personal, cultural, and powerful enough to change your body, how you think, and who you are as a person. This is because food contains information in the form of nutrients. Nutrients are the building blocks of your entire body, including cells, tissues, organs, and organ systems.[1] If you're eating nutritious food, your cells will be robust and healthy, leading to vibrant, whole body health. If you're eating highly refined foods that lack vitamins and minerals, then you are going to feel and look like it. However, you can transform your entire body just by changing your diet.

In this section, we will look at how nutrients affect your mind and body, the principles of healthy eating, cooking methods, personal and cultural food choices, and how to cultivate mindful eating practices.

NUTRIENTS

Have you ever craved a particular food? Your body is telling you it needs certain nutrients. Craving steak? You might need protein and iron. Are you craving fruit? You might need carbohydrates, water, vitamins, and minerals. Nutrients build every cell in your body, from brain, immune, skin, blood, and muscle cells. Without them, cells can't form properly or perform their functions, leading to trouble thinking, low immunity, fatigue, chronic inflammation, and increased chances of disease.[2]

Cells constantly undergo turnover and renewal, meaning new cells form when old cells die off. Some cells like skin cells are completely replaced within a month, while others like bone take years. Nutrition is a critical part of this process. Protein from your diet makes up the cell structure, fats comprise the cell membrane, carbohydrates provide energy, vitamins are essential for cellular metabolism, and minerals contribute to cell form and function. The process is compromised if your diet lacks any of these vital nutrients. If you feed your cells what they need, everything else falls into place. You'll feel better, look better, and think more clearly because your cells are strong and healthy.

Here's a short list of common nutrients we need to consume and where we can get them;

- **Vitamins**: Vitamins A, C, D, E, K and the B vitamins are important for various bodily functions. They are found in fruits, veggies, whole grains, dairy and lean meats.

- **Minerals**: Calcium, iron, magnesium, potassium, selenium, and zinc are important for the cells, enzymes and bodily processes. They're found in foods like dairy products, leafy greens, legumes, whole grains, and lean meats.

- **Fiber**: Supports gut health, aids digestion, is satiating, and helps regulate blood sugar levels. Sources include fruits, vegetables, whole grains, legumes, and nuts.

- **Water**: Essential for hydration and overall bodily functions. It's important to consume half your weight in ounces daily.

- **Antioxidants**: Beta-carotene, lycopene, resveratrol, flavonoids, polyphenols, and ECGC from green tea. Found in colorful fruits and vegetables, nuts, seeds, and certain spices and help protect your cells from damage caused by free radicals.

- **Omega-3 fatty acids**: Essential fatty acids important for brain health and reducing inflammation. Sources include fatty fish (like salmon and mackerel), flaxseeds, chia seeds, and walnuts.

- **Carbohydrates**: Provide energy and include sources like fruits, vegetables, whole grains, and legumes.

- **Proteins**: Essential for building and repairing tissues, found in foods such as meat, poultry, fish, dairy products, legumes, and plant-based sources like tofu and tempeh.

- **Fats**: Necessary for energy, hormone production, and nutrient absorption. Include sources like avocados, nuts, seeds, olive oil, and fatty fish and meats.

- **Probiotics**: Beneficial bacteria that support gut health. Found in fermented foods like yogurt, kefir, sauerkraut, and kimchi.

PRINCIPLES OF HEALTHY EATING

The food you eat can be either the safest and most powerful form of medicine or the slowest form of poison.

~ Ann Wigmore

Before we get into the principles of healthy eating, I want to remind you that there's no one right diet for everyone. Diet is very personal. Some of us need more protein and fat, while others do better with more carbohydrates. Some of us do fine eating sourdough bread and dairy, while others end up inflamed.

Someone may thrive on a vegan diet, while others completely fall apart. A nursing mother will likely need to eat more than her non-nursing female friends of the same age. A sedentary grandma will likely eat less than her growing athletic grandson.

Diet is also cultural and region-specific.[3] Someone living in Japan will likely have a different flavor palette than someone living in the Middle East. My German husband prefers traditional German food, while I, born and raised in Southern California, prefer the local cuisine. All of us can be equally healthy. So keep this in mind when you read the following sections, and don't get caught up thinking you have to change everything at once. You don't, nor would I recommend it. However, all of us can benefit from eating healthier, and every cuisine has healthy options. Even fast food restaurants have healthier options. Instead of ordering a burger, fries, and coke, you can order a burger lettuce wrapped or a chicken salad with unsweetened ice tea.

To change your habits around eating, start with one thing and work on that until it feels natural. I recommend picking the lowest-hanging fruit. In other words, choose what's easiest for you to change. When that becomes a habit, pick another thing and continue improving your diet in phases. Over time, you'll notice significant changes in your body.

BEING WELL

Now that we got that disclaimer out of the way, let me introduce you to what I believe are the fundamental principles of healthy eating;

1. Keep ultra-processed and inflammatory foods out of your diet.
2. Focus on real, whole foods in their natural or minimally processed form.
3. Eat primarily plants, preferably non-starchy vegetables.

These are the basics. If you can follow these simple principles, you'll be doing better than the average person. Below is a breakdown in more detail.

AVOID ULTRA-PROCESSED FOOD

If there's just one thing you're willing to do to improve your health by far, avoiding ultra-processed, inflammatory foods will have the most significant impact.[4] I'm not talking about a jar of tomato sauce or canned beans; Ultra-processed foods contain a list of ingredients that most people can't pronounce. These ingredients are chemicals that allow the food to be shelf-stable and full of flavor. They're molded into cute and conveniently sized shapes to appear more appetizing and faster eating. They include added dyes, preservatives, conditioners, stabilizers, artificial flavors, salt, sugar, and refined oils, all of which destroy your gut and beneficial flora, harming your digestion and immune system.[5] The following are examples of ultra-processed foods;

- Potato chips
- Sodas
- Processed meats
- Cookies
- Candy
- Cereals
- Margarine
- Shelf stable bread
- Instant noodles and ramen
- Frozen meals

The problem with ultra-processed food is that they're designed to be addicting, so you eat more and continue to buy the product. They are high in calories and low in nutrition, which is why so many people who eat ultra-processed foods are overweight. A study from 2019 found that people on a high ultra-processed diet overate by as much as 500 calories daily compared to when they were placed on a primarily unprocessed diet.[6]

Even products marketed as healthy and sold in health food stores can be ultra-processed and high in salt, sugar, and refined oils. Watch out for buzzwords with a healthy connotation, such as plant-based, gluten free, and keto. While they sound healthy, these foods can be highly processed. Read the label and skip it if it contains words you can't pronounce.

BEING WELL

Ultra-processed foods are not real food. They're convenient and taste good but are detrimental to your health.[7] Limit your intake as much as possible. If you focus on eating healthier foods with high fiber and water content that fill you up, you'll be less likely to reach for ultra-processed foods.

EAT MINIMALLY PROCESSED FOODS

On the other hand, minimally processed foods are excellent food choices. Compared to ultra-processed foods, they contain only a few recognizable ingredients and are often free from added sugar, salt, artificial additives, and unhealthy fats. Examples of minimally processed foods include;

- Frozen fruit & vegetables
- Plain yogurt & kefir
- Cheese
- Tofu & Tempeh
- Fermented vegetables
- Dried fruit
- Roasted seeds & nuts
- Canned beans, fish, or vegetables
- Tomato sauce
- Cold pressed oils such as olive, coconut, and avocado

EAT

In some cases, minimally processed foods can be healthier than their unprocessed counterparts. For example, yogurt and kefir are fermented dairy products that contain beneficial organisms that aid digestion and gut health. They also tend to be lower in lactose, a type of sugar from milk that many people can't digest.

EAT REAL FOOD

Real foods are whole foods such as vegetables, fruits, meats, fish, eggs, whole grains, legumes, beans, and dairy in their natural form. For example, this could include a baked sweet potato but not french fries. A pork chop, but not bacon. Whole grains but not a donut. A bone-in ribeye steak but not a Slim Jim. Corn on the cob but not chips. An apple but not apple pie.

Whole foods are healthy because they are nutrient-dense, meaning they are high in essential nutrients such as vitamins, minerals, fiber, and antioxidants relative to their calorie content. They help nourish the cells by providing nutrients that support various bodily functions, including growth, maintenance, and repair of tissues, as well as immune, energy, and cognitive functions.

When you consume whole foods, you're getting a diverse array of nutrients that work together synergistically. An example of nutrient synergy is spinach's iron and vitamin C. Iron from plants is not as absorbable as the kind found in animal products. However, vitamin C helps convert plant iron into a more absorbable form, increasing the body's ability to utilize it. Ultra-processed foods sometimes have nutrients added to them, but those nutrients are isolated and don't work together with other nutrients. It's much better to eat foods that naturally contain a mix of nutrients so they work together.

A benefit of whole plant foods is that they're high in water and fiber, so they tend to be satiating, promoting a sense of fullness and satisfaction, reducing the likelihood of overeating.

Finally, whole foods are more economical and sustainable than processed food. Packaged foods require more resources for production and disposal. Buying whole foods is the better choice for you and the planet.

EAT PRIMARILY PLANTS

Plant foods are associated with a lower risk for chronic diseases such as obesity, heart disease, type 2 diabetes, and certain cancers.[8, 9, 10] Whole plant foods are nutrient-dense, contain water which helps with hydration, and are high in antioxidants which help neutralize chemicals that damage cells. Plants contain fiber which feeds the good bacteria in your gut. When consumed alongside animal foods, fiber helps cholesterol exit the body through bowel movements. Regenerative, grass-fed and pasture raised animal products are nutrient-dense. When not overdone, they're incredibly healing and have their place in healthy diets.[11] Just be sure to eat them with plants such as in a big salad or with grilled veggies for better health.

EAT

BE VEGICURIOUS

When it comes to plants, variety is essential. The gut is home to trillions of microorganisms crucial to our overall health, including digestion, nutrient absorption, immune function, and mental well-being. These microbes thrive on a diversity of plant fibers.[12] The current recommendations are to aim to eat at least 30 different plant fibers a week to promote gut diversity.[13] While this may seem daunting, you might be eating more plant fibers than you think. Spices like ginger, turmeric, oregano, thyme, peppercorns, and other spices count. Just start where you are and work your way up at your own pace. Here are some examples of how to add more plant fibers to your diet;

- Buy various fruits, veggies, legumes, and whole grains, and eat them throughout the week.

- Aim to have a different vegetable with every meal.

- Make trail mix with various nuts, seeds, and dried fruit. I combine macadamia nuts, pistachios, walnuts, pumpkin seeds, dried cranberries, raisins, and blueberries. That's seven different plant fibers.

- Make smoothies with various fruits, veggies, nuts, seeds, and oats to make them creamy.

- Change up your whole grains and legumes daily. For example, one day, have brown rice and chickpea curry; the next, have quinoa and lentils with different spices. Then another day, have millet with black beans and peas.

BEING WELL

- Eat oatmeal for breakfast with various fruits, seeds, and nuts, or make it savory with broth and steamed veggies.
- Make a big pot of veggie soup with as many veggies, beans, and whole grains as possible.

The majority of a healthy meal should be non-starchy, deep-colored veggies. Think big salads with the proteins and fats of your choice, hearty vegetable soup with meatballs, steamed veggies with black rice and tofu, sautéed collard greens with 1/2 baked sweet potato and salmon, spaghetti squash with lentil bolognese sauce. The meal options are endless once you learn how to set up your plate.

Can you be healthy and be a strict vegan? The answer is yes, with a caveat; you'll have to think more about your food choices. It's much easier to become deficient on a vegan diet and overeat on starches and processed foods, but that doesn't mean you can't do it. Listen to your body, be mindful to eat enough proteins and healthy fats, take B12 and DHA supplements from algae, and go easy on ultra-processed plant foods.

IGNORE FAT-FREE PROPAGANDA

If you were around in the 80s, you probably remember the crusade against fat. It seemed like overnight everything in the grocery store had a fat-free label on it. I remember fat-free milk, yogurt, cereal, cookies, crackers, dips, chips, and salad dressing. Even naturally fat-free foods like ketchup proudly wore the fat-free label. The idea was that fat made you fat, and by avoiding it, you'd finally be able to fit into your skinny jeans and live happily ever after. Unfortunately, we all got fatter during that time.

According to the Center for Disease Control and Prevention (CDC), the average American is about 25 pounds heavier than before the fat-free revolution.[14] The problem is when you take out an entire macronutrient like fat, you end up replacing it with simple carbohydrates like sugar which cause insulin to spike. Insulin is the hormone that tells your body to store fat. Secondly, fat is satiating, and foods that lack fat tend to be less satisfying, so you end up eating more. Thirdly, all these fat-free products were ultra-processed. If you remember from the previous section, ultra-processed foods are calorie-rich, nutrient-poor, and designed to make you eat the entire package. While the rate of heart disease has gone down since the 1980s, the rate of diabetes has gone up.[15] We traded one chronic lifestyle disease for another.

It took decades to overturn that bad advice, and while that reign of terror isn't entirely over, we now know it's more about the type and quality of fat rather than the entire macronutrient. Good fats are incredibly healing. They provide energy, are involved in hormone regulation and synthesis, indirectly balance insulin, build the cell membrane, and help in the absorption of fat soluble vitamins A, D, E, and K.[16] You need fat in your diet. You just have to know which ones to eat, and which ones to avoid.

BEING WELL

EAT HEALTHY FATS

Most of your fat intake should be from whole foods in their natural, unprocessed forms such as avocados, almonds, macadamia nuts, hazelnuts, and omega-3 from fish.[17] These foods have a healthy ratio of omega-3 to omega-6 fatty acids and contain other nutrients that absorb well with fat. Minimally processed oils such as extra virgin olive oil, coconut, and avocado are healthy choices and make good cooking oils.[17] Here's a list of good fat options;

- **Avocados** are rich in heart-healthy monounsaturated fats, are nutrients dense and high in antioxidants, help blood sugar regulation, and are anti-inflammatory.

- **Fatty fish** such as wild-caught salmon, mackerel, and sardines are excellent sources of anti-inflammatory omega-3 fatty acids, can lower triglycerides, and support brain and eye health.

- **Eggs** are nutrient-dense, high in healthy fats like monounsaturated and omega-3 fatty acids, rich in choline, essential for brain function, and high in antioxidants.

- **Nuts & seeds** are nutrient-dense, full of heart-healthy monounsaturated and polyunsaturated fats, are associated with a lower risk of heart disease, and promote healthy weight.

- **Olives** are a good source of heart-healthy monounsaturated fats, contain various antioxidants, are anti-inflammatory, and help with weight management.

EAT

- **Coconut** is a good source of medium chain triglycerides (MCTs), which provide energy, improve cognitive function, and promote fullness, helping with weight management.

- **Organic full-fat dairy from grass-fed cows** is nutrient-dense, assists with calcium absorption and bone health, is associated with a lower risk of type 2 diabetes, and contains saturated, monounsaturated, and polyunsaturated fats. Eat in moderation.

- **Grass-fed meats** are nutrient-dense and high in antioxidants, are lower in fat than conventionally raised animal products, have a favorable balance of omega-3 to omega-6 fatty acid ratio, and contain conjugated linoleum acid (CLA), saturated, and monounsaturated fats.

- **Omega-3 fatty acids** are found in fatty fish, walnuts, and seeds like flax, chia, and hemp. They are necessary for the heart, brain, eyes, joints, pregnancy, and early development. Omega-3 fatty acids reduce inflammation.

- **Extra virgin olive oil (EVOO)** is a minimally processed oil high in antioxidants. It's good for the heart, brain, and microbiome. EVOO is anti-inflammatory and promotes healthy weight.

AVOID UNHEALTHY FATS

Vegetable oils also known as seed oils, such as soybean, canola, corn, cottonseed, sunflower, and safflower should be avoided in your diet. These oils are heavily refined, bleached, and deodorized. They tend to be high in omega-6 fatty acids, which, when consumed in excess, throw off the delicate ratio of omega-3 to omega-6 fatty acids. The health problems associated with vegetable oils are no joke; cardiovascular disease, cancer, obesity, inflammation and chronic inflammatory conditions, oxidative stress and cellular damage, and impaired nutrient absorption.[18, 19]

Restaurants are notorious for cooking with these oils because they're cheap and lack strong flavors due to processing. Out of all the vegetable oils, canola is thought to be the best option because it has a better ratio of omega-3 to omega-6. However, the omega-3s in canola are easily damaged and oxidized due to high temperatures during processing.[20] If you do consume canola make sure it's cold pressed. Personally I still avoid canola and cook with fats such as butter, extra virgin olive, coconut, and avocado oils.

Hydrogenated fats are vegetable oils that have had hydrogen added during processing, extending their shelf life and making them solid at room temperature. Food manufacturers commonly use partially hydrogenated fats in ultra-processed foods such as margarine, baked goods, chips, and microwave popcorn. Restaurants use them as an oil for deep frying and baking. You'll find them in fried foods; french fries, fried chicken, doughnuts, and fried snacks. Partially hydrogenated fats sound like the better option, but they are not. Partially hydrogenated fats contain trans fats associated with heart disease, stroke, type 2 diabetes, inflammation, obesity, and decreased cognitive function.[21, 22] Don't buy foods with hydrogenated or partially hydrogenated fats. Read labels, and if an ingredient contains the word hydrogenated, put it back on the shelf.

Eat These Fats	Not These Fats
Avocado	Refined seed & vegetable oil
Fatty Fish	Soybean oil
Eggs	Corn oil
Seeds	Cottonseed oil
Nuts	Sunflower oil
Olives	Safflower oil
Full fat dairy	Margarine
Grass-fed meats	Hydrogenated oil
Extra virgin olive oil	Trans fat
Omega-3	Shortening

KNOW THE SMOKING POINTS

When cooking with fat, you need to consider its smoking point. Smoking points refer to the temperature that food starts to break down and produce smoke. When fats reach their smoking points, they create toxic compounds such as acrolein, acrylamides, and polycyclic aromatic hydrocarbons (PAHs).[23] These compounds are associated with various health problems, including inflammation, oxidative stress, cellular damage, the formation of free radicals, and certain

BEING WELL

cancers.[23] High heat also degrades certain heat-sensitive nutrients and can leave your food tasting burnt. Each fat has a smoking point. It's better to use fats with high smoking points when cooking at high temperatures. For example, avocado oil, coconut oil, and ghee all have high smoking points and are good choices for stir-frying. Roasting and baking are generally done between 300-400 degrees Fahrenheit, so the above oils as well as olive oil and butter can be good options. Oils such as flaxseed, walnut, hemp, and pumpkin break down at low temperatures and should never be used to cook with. These oils are best drizzled over salads or other foods. Here's a table of approximate smoking points of oils from highest to lowest;

Cooking fat	Smoking point F	Smoking point C
Avocado oil	520	271
Ghee	450-485	232-251
Tallow	400-420	204-215
Coconut oil	400-450	204-232
Lard	370-400	188-204
Butter	350-375	177-191
Olive oil	375-420	191-215
EVOO	325-375	163-191
Flax oil	225	107

EAT

EAT THE RAINBOW

Mother Nature really did try to make getting nutrients easy. She color-coded our food, hung them low on trees and bushes, and gave them enticing scents and flavors. By eating a variety of colorful fruits and vegetables, you're on your way to getting a broad spectrum of health-promoting compounds. Phytonutrients, the nutrients found mostly in plants, contain pigments of different colors. These colors are clues to a food's unique nutrient profile and are correlated with lower risks of disease and mortality.[24] Aim to eat foods from each color group several times a week. Here's a breakdown of colors and the nutrients associated with them;

- **Red foods** contain essential nutrients such as anthocyanins, lycopene, and vitamins A and C. These include tomatoes, red bell peppers, strawberries, watermelon, cherries, and cranberries.

- **Orange foods** are rich in beta-carotene, vitamin C, fiber, potassium, vitamin B6, and antioxidants. These include carrots, mangos, sweet potatoes, pumpkin, butternut squash, oranges, apricots, and turmeric.

- **Yellow foods** contain vitamins A, C, folate, and potassium. These include bananas, yellow bell peppers, corn, squash, pineapple, and ginger.

- **Green foods** contain vitamins K, C, folate, minerals, fiber, and phytonutrients like chlorophyll and lutein. They include broccoli, cilantro, parsley, spinach, kale, leafy greens, green cabbage, peas, edamame, seaweed,

51

okra, Brussels sprouts, green beans, and avocados. Eat green foods daily.

- **Blue/Purple foods** contain anthocyanins, vitamins C, K, and fiber. They include blueberries, blackberries, purple grapes, eggplant, and purple cabbage.

- **Brown foods** contain fiber, essential fatty acids, various B vitamins, and minerals. They include whole grains, legumes, lentils, chickpeas, nuts, and seeds.

- **Black foods** contain anthocyanins, polyphenols, iron, potassium, fiber, vitamins C and K, various B vitamins, and healthy fats. They include black varieties of rice, beans, lentils, tea, sesame seeds, and quinoa.

- **White foods** contain fiber, potassium, and vitamin C. White foods include napa cabbage, radish, turnips, parsnips, cauliflower, mushrooms, onions, garlic, white beans, apples, and pears.

Don't be fooled by colorful processed foods; they do not contain phytonutrients. They contain chemicals to enhance their appearance and make them fun for children to eat. Research has associated several food colorings with health problems.[25] Red dye #40 may cause allergic reactions such as hives, itching, difficulty breathing, hyperactivity and behavioral changes in children, and cancer.[26] Yellow dye #5 can cause allergic reactions and hyperactivity in children.[27] Yellow dye #6 led to animals developing tumors in animal studies. Blue dyes #1 and #2 may cause hyperactivity in children.[28] Studies suggest green dye #3 causes tumors in animal laboratory studies.

EAT

DRINK MORE WATER

Nancy came into my office with fatigue, trouble concentrating, headaches, and low back pain. Her doctor told her it was perimenopause and sent her on her way. Frustrated by his response, she came to see if I could help. I did an assessment and noticed her tongue, mouth, eyes, and skin were all dry. I performed the skin turgor test, where you pinch the skin on the back of the hand, hold it for a second, then release it. Well-hydrated skin immediately snaps back, while dehydrated skin moves slowly, often resulting in a "tenting" appearance. Her skin tented, a clear sign of dehydration.

I asked how many cups of water she drank during the day, to which she replied, some when she remembers but usually drinks iced tea instead. She also drank coffee every morning and alcohol on the weekends, both dehydrating.

I told her all of her symptoms could be due to dehydration and to drink a full glass of water as soon as she wakes up every morning. I also advised her to drink at least half her weight in ounces of water daily, to focus on eating hydrating foods such as cucumbers, watermelon, salads, strawberries, spinach, celery, and coconut water, and to cut back on coffee, alcohol, and iced tea. She was baffled that it could be so simple, but she did what I advised, and when I saw her a week later, all of her symptoms were gone.

People often overlook the healing powers of water. Water is the universal solvent, capable of combining with everything in its environment. It is the vehicle that transports nutrients, hormones, neurotransmitters, and waste products throughout the body. Every second, billions of chemical reactions occur in the body, all in a water medium. Without water, these reactions can't take place. Signs of dehydration include dry mouth, fatigue, headaches, dizziness, constipation, increased thirst, muscle cramps, irritability, dark colored urine, and trouble concentrating.[29]

Benefits of water include;

- Keeping the muscles, joints, and other tissues well-fed and lubricated.[30]

- Improving digestion by helping dissolve nutrients, soften stools, and prevents constipation.[29]

- Aiding in weight management by promoting feelings of fullness as well as supporting metabolism and the breakdown of fat.[31]

- Supporting detoxification by helping to remove waste and toxins from the body.[32]

- Improving energy by transporting essential nutrients like glucose and oxygen to cells.[29]

- Regulating temperature by preventing the body from overheating.[29]

But not all water is created equal. Water absorbs and mixes with everything in its environment. While most public water systems meet US safety standards, tap water still contains pharmaceuticals and other chemicals, such as endocrine-disrupting compounds (EDC). If you're drinking tap water, you may be consuming high levels of chemicals without knowing it. I highly recommend drinking filtered water. Here are my recommendations around drinking water;

- Drink a full glass of water when you wake up to flush out metabolic waste and start your day hydrated.

- Drink at least half your body weight of water in ounces. For example, if you weigh 200 pounds, drink 100 ounces of water daily. If you're nowhere near that amount, then work your way up. Add more and more each day until you reach your recommended amount.

- Add a squeeze of lemon or lime to your water for added electrolytes. Add a pinch of sea salt for trace minerals.

- Sip your water slowly throughout the day. You don't want to gulp it down because it will move too quickly through the stomach and not get absorbed by the cells.

- Consume foods naturally high in water such as fruits and vegetables. Fruit and vegetable smoothies are hydrating and a good way to get your plant fibers in.

- Bring water in a glass or stainless steel container with you whenever you leave the house.

- Limit or eliminate caffeine and alcohol intake. Both have a diuretic effect which can lead to dehydration. Drink a full glass of water before consuming caffeine or alcohol.

- If you're craving sweets, are tired, or have a headache, drink a glass or two of water, then see how you feel.

- Hydrate before, during, and after exercise.

BEING WELL

- Choose a filtration system that filters out pharmaceuticals and endocrine-disrupting compounds. Be sure to maintain it and replace the filters according to manufacturer recommendations.
- If you get a reverse osmosis filter, add minerals back into your water.
- Pay attention to your body's cues. If you're thirsty, have dry skin, or dark-colored urine, you're dehydrated and need to drink more fluids.

Water is essential for life. Ensuring you're properly hydrated can transform your health, energy levels, and overall well-being.

BE MINDFUL OF PORTION SIZES

Portion sizes have grown significantly over the years thanks to food industry marketing and pretty packaging, larger plates and bowls, and the reliance on eating out and takeout culture. Larger portion sizes have become socially acceptable. However, there are many reasons why you want to keep your portion sizes reasonable. Besides weight gain, people who regularly overeat suffer from blood sugar imbalances leading to energy slumps and fatigue. Overeating also causes digestive issues such as bloating, indigestion, acid reflux, and heartburn. Overeating can lead to nutritional imbalances, problems regulating the appetite, disordered eating patterns,

EAT

and feelings of guilt and shame related to food and body image.

How can we calculate the right portion size? Portion size is dependable on the individual's age, gender, activity level, hunger level, nutritional status, and whether or not they're pregnant or nursing. However, I've provided some general guidelines on portion sizes for you to follow. You may need more or less depending on your unique nutritional needs.

- **Protein** such as meat, fish, tofu, poultry, beans or legumes should be about the size of the palm of your hand, minus your fingers.

- **Non-starchy vegetables** such as broccoli, leafy greens, asparagus, cauliflower, cabbage, and carrots should fill at least half your plate.

- **Grains & starchy vegetables** like quinoa, brown rice, pasta, sweet potatoes or squash should be limited to a fist-sized amount.

- **Fruit** should also be limited to a fist-sized portion.

- **Fats** can be measured out using the size of your thumb.

Smaller plates can help keep portions at reasonable amounts. Again this is just a guide; your unique nutritional needs depend on many factors.

EAT AT REGULAR TIMES

There are many meal timing strategies, but most people benefit from spacing their meals four hours apart. The reason for this is when we eat; the body secretes digestive enzymes and stomach acid that break down food and nutrients so they can get absorbed into the bloodstream. This takes time, and eating too frequently disrupts the process leading to digestive issues such as indigestion, gas, bloating, and abdominal pain. Snacking can also lead to energy crashes and mood swings due to unstable blood sugar levels.[33]

Another cool thing about digestion is that the muscles in our intestines contract in cyclical waves between meals and when we're sleeping. This is called the Migrating Motility Complex (MMC), and takes about 90 minutes to kick in. The contractions move food particles, bacteria, and debris along the digestive tract, helping maintain a healthy gut environment. If you're constantly snacking, this process gets interrupted, increasing the risk of bacteria overgrowth, bloating, and abdominal pain.[34] Spacing meals four hours apart gives the MMC enough time to do its job.

In general, you want to stop eating three hours before sleeping. Digestion requires energy and increases body temperature, heart rate, and metabolism, leading to poor sleep.[34] Eating too close to bed can also cause the stomach's contents to move up the GI tract into the throat. This is called acid reflux or heartburn and can happen when we lie down due to gravity.

Give your body time to digest your food before lying down to sleep.

SHRINK YOUR EATING WINDOW

Your eating window starts when you first eat or drink something with calories and ends when you finish eating for the day. So, if you generally start breakfast at 8 am and finish eating dinner by 6 pm, you have a 10-hour eating window. A 10-hour eating window gives your body about 14 hours of rest between meals. The recommended eating window is 12 hours or less. Research shows it can help with many things, including weight loss, improved insulin sensitivity, cellular repair, brain health, reduced inflammation, longevity, and disease prevention.[35, 36, 37]

Calculate your usual eating window. If it's more than 12 hours, I recommend scaling back your eating window by 1/2 hour each day until you reach 12 hours. However, if you have hypoglycemia, this is not recommended. Get your blood sugar regulated first before you change your eating window.

Here's a recap of what we just went over;

- Space your meals four hours apart.
- Stop eating three hours before going to bed.
- Keep your eating window 12 hours or less.

CHOOSE HEALTHIER COOKING METHODS

A friend of mine once invited me over for what she said was going to be a healthy meal full of vegetables. Turns out she deep fried all of the veggies and served them over white rice with a surgery sauce. I didn't have the heart to tell her deep frying destroyed all of the nutrients, created cancer causing compounds, and turned the veggies into a vehicle of rancid fats. That would have been mean.

But this brings up a good point—how you cook your food can either make nutrients easier to absorb or completely wipe them out. While some foods like leafy greens, citrus fruits, berries, nuts, and seeds are better for you raw, most foods are better when lightly cooked due to enhanced digestibility and nutrient availability. Here's a breakdown of cooking methods in the order of healthiest to least healthiest;

- **Steaming** is the healthiest of all cooking methods. It breaks down food structures so nutrients are extracted but not destroyed. Steaming retains most of the food's flavor and texture without adding extra fat.

- **Dehydrating** uses warm air to gently remove the water content in food, killing off microorganisms while extending shelf life. It's an excellent cooking method because it concentrates flavors, preserves most nutrients except for water soluble ones, and reduces the risk of food-borne illness.

- **Poaching** uses liquids such as water or broth to cook food gently at low temperatures. It retains a lot of nutrition and flavor, making it a desired cooking method for eggs, chicken, and fish.

- **Slow cooking** involves cooking food at low temperatures for an extended period. Slow cooking retains nutrients because it cooks the food at low temperatures.

- **Pressure cooking** uses steam and pressure to cook food. Pressure cooking is quick and helps the food retain nutrients.

- **Grilling** involves cooking over an open flame, allowing excess fat to drip off. It's great for meats, fish, chicken, veggies, and fruit like pineapple. However, grilled food can quickly become toxic when charred or burned. Avoid this by precooking in an oven to minimize time on the grill.

- **Baking & Roasting** both use dry heat to cook food. Baking at lower temperatures will help to retain nutrients as well as enhance the flavor without having to add fat. High temperatures and long cooking times can destroy nutrients, so keep the temperatures low and cooking times short.

- **Stir-frying** is not as healthy as the above methods because the heat is generally higher. However, cooking time is shorter, which can help preserve nutrients. Choose healthy cooking oils such as avocado and coconut, which have higher smoking points.

- **Sautéing** is similar to stir-frying and can be a semi-healthy cooking option due to the shorter cooking time.

However, like stir-frying, sauté at the lowest temperature possible to achieve the desired effect and use healthy cooking oils such as avocado or coconut.

- **Boiling** loses a lot of nutrients because the high heat causes them to leach out of the food into the water. Use less water and shorter cooking times to minimize nutrient loss. You can also consume the liquid or use it in other recipes.

- **Microwaving** is fast, convenient, and retains nutrients because it uses shorter cooking times.[38] It also requires little to no extra fats. However, you need to be mindful of using microwave-safe containers. Do not microwave your food in plastic because plastic particles leach out into your food.[39] Glass is the best option.

- **Deep-frying** is extremely unhealthy.[40] The high temperatures and cooking oils destroy heat-sensitive nutrients. Deep fried foods absorb a great deal of cooking oil making them high in calories and unhealthy fats. They contain harmful compounds such as advanced glycation end-producers (AGEs), acrylamides, and polycyclic aromatic hydrocarbons (PAHs). These compounds are linked to inflammation, oxidative stress, advanced aging, and disease.[22] Don't deep-fry your food!

EAT

AVOID PESTICIDES

One of the most underrated topics in health is the amount of chemicals added to our foods. The use of synthetic pesticides and herbicides such as glyphosate, started in the early 1900s with the advancement of industrial agriculture to increase production. Unfortunately, various health problems are associated with pesticides, including;

- **Neurological disorders** such as Parkinson's disease and developmental disorders in children.[41]

- **Cancers** such as leukemia, lymphoma, and prostate cancer.[42]

- **Endocrine disorders** such as hormone imbalances, reproductive issues, and developmental problems.[43]

- **Immune conditions** such as allergies, sensitivities, and respiratory problems.[44]

To decrease your exposure to pesticides, herbicides, and other chemicals in your food;

- **Choose organic whenever possible:** Foods with the organic label have undergone a rigorous certification process and do not contain synthetic pesticides. Yes, organic foods are more expensive. But you either pay higher prices for your food now, or higher healthcare costs to manage lifestyle diseases later. On a side note, using genetically modified organisms (GMOs) is strictly prohibited in organic products.

- **Wash and peel produce:** Thoroughly wash and peel your produce to remove any pesticide residues on the surface.

- **Grow your food:** Use organic seeds and plants to grow your own food.

- **Support local farmers:** Many local farmers use sustainable farming practices. Speaking directly with farmers can help you learn about their methods.

- **Cooking methods:** Certain cooking methods such as baking, roasting, and stir-frying can help break down pesticide residues.

- **Diversity:** Consume a diverse range of foods to minimize exposure to a single chemical.

- **Dirty Dozen:** Consult the Environmental Working Group's (EWG) website that publishes the "Dirty Dozen" annually, a list of the foods most heavily sprayed with pesticides. They also publish the "Clean Fifteen," a list of the least sprayed foods. **https://www.ewg.org/foodnews/about.php**

BUY ANTIBIOTIC & HORMONE FREE MEATS

In the 1940s, farmers began using antibiotics in livestock to treat infections in poultry. Since then, the use of antibiotics in animal products has increased significantly. While it has undoubtedly reduced disease-related loss, the use of antibiotics in animal products has harmed our health in many ways, including;

- The rise of antibiotic-resistant bacteria and the transfer of antibiotic-resistant genes led to difficult-to-treat human infections.[43]
- Changes to the animal's microbiome led to changes in the food products derived from these animals.[45]
- Some studies suggest children who consume animal products treated with antibiotics early in life may be at higher risk for developing allergies and sensitivities.[46]

To avoid unnecessary antibiotic exposure from animal products, look for labels that say "antibiotic-free" or "raised-without-antibiotics." Organic animal products are generally considered antibiotic free. Grass-fed, pasture-raised, and regeneratively raised animals are less likely to be treated with antibiotics than conventionally raised animals. Speak to the farmers to learn about their farming practices. Minimizing your consumption of animal products is another way to limit your exposure to antibiotics.

And don't think you're doing yourself a favor by eating meat with added hormones. Hormones added to food could disrupt the delicate balance of hormones in your body.[47] Eating food with added hormones can cause unwanted weight gain, fertility problems, cancer, acne, heart disease, and diabetes. Choose products that say "hormone-free" or "no hormones added."

BEING WELL

PREP YOUR MEALS

The best way to change your habits around food is by making healthy eating fun, easy, and accessible while making eating unhealthy food hard. How can you achieve this? Flood your fridge and pantry with healthy, whole, and minimally processed foods. Pack your freezer with frozen fruits, veggies, proteins, and single servings of homemade meals. Fill your fridge with fresh fruits, veggies, eggs, proteins, legumes, nut butter, healthy sauces, salsa, fermented veggies, milk, plain yogurts, cheese, and homemade meals. Stock your pantry with whole grains, oatmeal, and sourdough bread (if you eat them), canned tomato sauce, legumes, veggies, olives, tuna, salmon, broth, seaweed, nuts, seeds, dried fruit, sweet potatoes, spices, healthy oils like olive, avocado, and coconut. Put a bowl filled with fresh fruit on your kitchen counter for easy access.

Don't buy ultra-processed foods. If you have chips and cookies in your house, I guarantee you will eat them. If you don't, then you can't eat them. It's as simple as that. It's easier to avoid temptations when they're not around than to resist the ones in front of you. If you want a cookie, make a batch using any of the healthy ingredients mentioned above.

Yes, ultra-processed foods are convenient and save time. All you have to do is open up a package and start eating. But prepping food beforehand makes eating healthy just as convenient but much better for you. Pick a day to shop and meal prep so you have quick and healthy options throughout the week. Here are some meal prep ideas;

EAT

- **Eggs:** Make enough hard-boiled eggs to last your household a few days. Then add to sandwiches, salads, make egg salad, or eat as is with salt and pepper.

- **Baked Veggies:** Chop up a bunch of veggies and bake at 350 - 375 F for an hour with the seasoning of your choice. Then add them to your meals during the week.

- **Proteins:** Bake a bunch of chicken, turkey, pork, fish, tofu, or legumes to last your household a few days. Add cooked proteins to almost anything, including soups, salads, sandwiches, tacos, etc.

- **Fresh Veggies:** Slice up a bunch of veggies and put them in jars so when you're hungry, you can snack on them as is, dip them in hummus or guacamole, add them to salads, put them in sandwiches, or have as a side to your meal.

- **Protein Salads:** Make a batch of tuna, salmon, chicken, or bean salad using healthy fats like organic plain yogurt or avocados, and diced veggies like carrots, onions, and celery. You can eat it as is or put it on a salad or a sandwich.

- **Soup:** Make a giant pot of veggie soup, put it in individual containers, and freeze or keep it in the fridge. For a quick meal, reheat and eat it as is, or add some sliced baked chicken or garbanzo beans. If you have a few minutes to kick it up, spice it up with whatever you want. For example, if you're craving Mexican, add salsa, sliced avocado, cilantro, and chopped red onion. Add tamari, ginger shavings, and a splash of toasted sesame oil if you're craving Japanese. If you're craving Thai, add coconut milk and Thai curry paste. If you're craving Chile, add beans, ground beef, tomato paste, chili powder, cumin, paprika, garlic powder, onion powder, oregano, and cayenne pepper. You can even make it Indian by adding curry powder and lentils.

- **Salad:** Prepare a large salad that you can divide into different containers. I usually chop up a head of romaine, carrots, cucumbers, radishes, or whatever veggies I have on hand. Then when I'm hungry, I throw some sliced chicken or canned wild-caught salmon on it, nuts and seeds or sliced avocado, a couple of tablespoons of sauerkraut or kimchi, and a splash of olive oil and apple cider vinegar, or whatever homemade dressing I have on hand.

- **Rice:** Make a pot of rice. To keep things simple, you can reheat the rice with your protein, add some sauce and eat it as is or with a salad. If you have extra time, stir-fry rice with chopped veggies, eggs, protein, tamari, and a splash of toasted sesame oil. Or cook it with whatever spices you want.

- **Dressings:** Homemade dressings are so easy to make. A good ratio is 1:1 oil to acid. You can change this up according to the taste and consistency that you prefer. A simple oil and vinegar recipe is 1:1 oil to vinegar, 1 - 2 garlic cloves, a dash of mustard, and blend with salt and pepper. For a vegan Caesar salad recipe, I do 1/4th cup olive oil, 1/4th cup lemon juice, one tablespoon of hemp heart, one tablespoon of capers, and a couple cloves of garlic. Blend on high with salt and pepper until creamy.

EAT

- **Trail mix:** The options are endless here. Mix a bunch of nuts, seeds, and dried fruit. You can buy trail mix already made but be mindful not to purchase ones with added oils or sugar.

- **Snacks:** For something crunchy and salty, bake garbanzo beans or kale chips

- Keep it simple by having a hard-boiled egg with sliced avocado on toast topped with bagel seasoning and pickled onions (or no toast if you're grain free; I promise, over time, you won't miss the bread).

- Bake enough sweet potatoes to last a few days in the fridge. When you're hungry, grab one and reheat it. Add some butter, and you have a super delicious and filling snack. Add some lettuce on the side with beans or protein to make it a meal.

- For a very filling and quick meal, add one hard-boiled egg, a slice of cheese, a handful of nuts, and half an avocado on a bed of greens topped with a dressing of your choice.

- Make a charcuterie-style dinner with lots of little yummies like sliced proteins, cheese, eggs, pates, bread, salted nuts, olives, fresh and dried fruit, pickles, carrot sticks, celery sticks, lettuce, tomato, hummus, and guacamole.

Your options are endless once you learn how to meal prep. You can whip up all these meals quickly with minimal effort.

DON'T OVERCOMPLICATE IT

Sometimes we feel we have to make every meal a royal fest with lots of ingredients. We don't. And to be honest, my family doesn't care if I spend two hours cooking or two minutes. So don't complicate things. A healthy meal can be as simple as scrambled eggs with rice and veggies and sliced fruit for desert. My kids love baked chicken with rice and veggies. I know it can be challenging if you're a working single Mom. Ask for help and go easy on yourself. If you have to buy fast and ultra-processed food, get the least evil one you can afford.

ENJOY YOUR FOOD

Finally, there's a ton of flexibility when it comes to healthy eating, so please don't be intimidated by all the above information. I know it's a lot, but there are many healthy food options for you to explore and enjoy. Eating shouldn't be boring, and we all don't have to eat the same diet to be healthy. We all have different food preferences inspired by many factors, including what we ate as a child, the culture we grew up in, and our personal preferences. Each of us can be eating healthier so start with changing one food habit at a time.

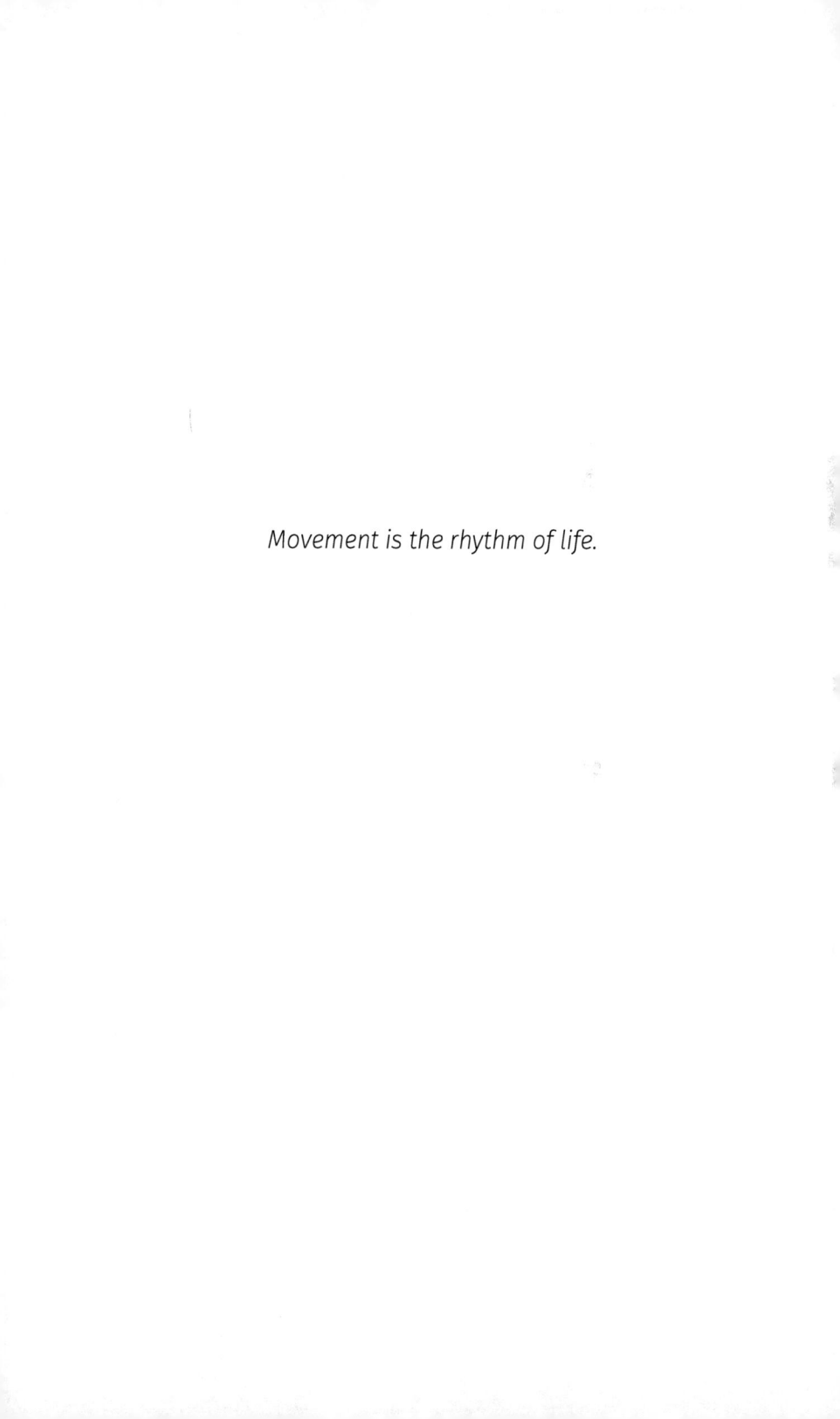

Movement is the rhythm of life.

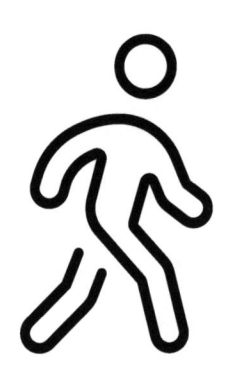

Move

If exercise were a pill, it would be the most widely prescribed medicine in the world.

~ Unknown

If you've ever felt insecure about starting a fitness journey, you're not alone. It's intimidating, especially at places like the gym where super fit people hang out and pump iron. Little old me feels silly waiting my turn, then moving the pin that holds the weights from near the bottom to the very first weight. I've thought to myself, do I even belong here?

But movement isn't just about looking good in your skinny jeans. It's about becoming the best version of yourself possible. It's about lowering your chances of dying from a heart attack, stroke, or cancer.[1, 2, 3] It's about not having to take medication for the rest of your life to manage diabetes, high blood pressure, or cholesterol.[4, 5, 6] It's about lowering your chances of becoming obese or ending up with a neurodegenerative disease like Alzheimer's, where you no longer recognize your loved ones.[7,8]

Movement is about feeling good with fewer bouts of depression or anxiety, it's about sleeping better, having more energy, thinking more clearly, experiencing better digestion, and becoming more robust and resilient to getting sick.[9,10,11,12,13] It's about twisting the lid off the jar of tomato sauce without spraining your wrist, lifting that box over your head without breaking your back, and sitting down and standing up without using your hands. Exercising is about maintaining independence, especially as you grow old into your golden years.

I don't want to spend the last years of my life having strangers take care of me because I lost the ability to take care of myself. Yes, while all of us have different genetics and life circumstances that could lead us down this path, most of us can do something about it, prolonging the time we have to do things for ourselves and possibly even prevent losing our independence in the first place. Exercise is about prevention, maintenance, and improvement, and it's never too late to start.

The best part is; movement doesn't have to be complicated or boring. You don't have to go to the gym and pump iron if that's not your calling. You have so many options available to you. Some won't even feel like exercising because you have so much fun doing them. But you do need to do something to preserve your strength, agility, and cardiovascular health. No one gets a free ride here. So what can you do?

MOVE

WHERE TO START

Start anywhere. Like anything else, the first step is just starting. Put on your shoes and go for a short walk around the block at home or on your lunch break. Bring a friend or your pet along to keep you company. You can go for a bike ride, a hike on an easy trail, swim, play sports with friends or family, go dancing, do yoga, take the stairs, or do some gardening which is surprisingly a physically demanding activity. Even cleaning the house is considered light exercise, especially when vacuuming or mopping.

If you're just starting out, think about what you like to do that comes naturally. Do you like nature? Then you'll probably enjoy outdoor activities like hiking, biking, or running. Do you like being around people or feel more motivated when you have an instructor? Then you might like taking classes like yoga, pilates, Zumba, spinning, boxing, TRX, etc. Are you competitive? Then you might enjoy playing tennis, pickleball, basketball, etc. Even ping pong is a fantastic form of movement because it burns calories, builds muscle, and improves cardiovascular health, hand-eye coordination, and reflexes.

Start small and try a few activities to find what you like. Remember, this isn't a competition—it's about becoming a better version of yourself. Set realistic goals and be patient. Don't just look at the scale to track your progress; think about how you feel overall, including your mood, sleep, energy levels, and ability to think more clearly. These are all markers of health and longevity.

HOW MUCH DO YOU NEED?

Surprisingly not that much. The recommended amount of movement is about 150 minutes of moderate aerobic or 75 minutes of vigorous activity weekly.[14] That comes down to about 21.4 of moderate or 10.7 minutes of vigorous aerobic activity daily. It's also advised to add in 20 minutes of muscle-strengthening activities twice weekly. That's it. And yet, many of us aren't even getting in the minimum recommended amount of movement per week. There are many reasons, but it boils down to this—modern life isn't conducive to movement. It has us cooped up in an office for long hours during the day. When we get home at night, we sit down and watch screens to unwind from our long days. If you're lucky, you'll do something active on the weekend, but unfortunately, most people spend their leisure time indoors playing video games or watching screens.

WHAT'S THE BEST KIND OF EXERCISE?

The best kind of exercise is whatever you like and are willing to do consistently. It also depends on your fitness level and health goals. One thing is for sure if you don't move, you won't get the benefits. You'd be surprised how many people forget this minor detail. So start small and make it fun so your brain associates exercise with doing what you love. Vary it up and aim to get exercise from the four main areas of fitness: 1)

Aerobic exercises, 2) muscle strength and endurance, 3) flexibility and agility, and 4) balance and coordination.

Aerobic Conditioning: Activities like brisk walking, running, cycling, dancing, and hiking get your heart rate up, increase blood flow, and delivers fresh oxygen to muscles.[15] Aerobic activities are good for your heart, lungs, and circulatory system and help you maintain a healthy weight. They're broken down into low, moderate, and vigorous intensity and are suitable for everyone regardless of physical abilities or age. Low-intensity activity includes leisurely walking, tai chi, stretching, cleaning the house, light gardening, and washing the car. Moderate-intensity activities include hiking, swimming, jogging, brisk walking, dancing, and biking. Vigorous-intensity activities include running, biking uphill, jumping jacks, and high-intensity interval training (HIIT).

Strength Training & Endurance: Strength training and endurance exercises, such as weight lifting, push-ups, lunges, and resistance bands, help to build and maintain muscle and strength, generate force and the ability to hold that force, and can help prevent injuries.[16] Everyone needs to do strength training exercises since we naturally lose muscle mass as we age. Strength training preserves muscle mass, increases bone density, improves metabolism, helps to maintain balance and stability, and allows older adults to maintain independence when performing basic activities of daily living.

Flexibility & Agility: Flexibility refers to the range of motion around a single or group of joints. Exercises such as yoga, tai chi, pilates, and stretching increase your range of motion and improve posture.[17] Agility is the ability to change directions quickly and easily, including speed, reaction time, and coordination. Agility exercises focus on fast, sharp direction changes, footwork, and reaction times. Agility exercises include box jumps, t-drills, lateral hops, and shuttle runs. Both flexibility and agility exercises focus on functional fitness, which aims to improve your ability to perform daily activities safely and efficiently.

Balance & Coordination: Balance exercises are essential for your brain and require knowing where your body is in space. Balance exercises include balancing on one foot or walking heel to toe with closed eyes. Coordination refers to your ability to smoothly and efficiently coordinate your movements. It requires good timing and the ability to use your muscles. Both balance and coordination exercises improve posture, increase core strength, improve focus and concentration, and are crucial for preventing falls as you age.[18]

As mentioned above, aim to do 150 minutes of moderate or 75 minutes of vigorous exercise weekly. You can do the recommended amount in one session, say a 2.5-hour hike, or in shorter 30-minute sessions five days a week. Also, include at least two 20-minute strength training sessions that work all the muscle groups every week. Don't be afraid to mix it up and have fun.

The following is a short list of popular exercises for those just getting started on their fitness journey.

WALKING

Walking might be the most natural form of exercise for humans. It's something we've been doing for 200,000 years as a species, and most of us since around the age of one. You don't even have to think about it. Put one foot in front of the other, then switch and you're walking. Walking improves cardiovascular health by increasing heart rate and circulation, and lowering blood pressure and cholesterol levels. It can help you stay at an optimal weight or lose weight when combined with a healthy diet. Walking is gentle on the joints, improves mood and reduces stress and anxiety. It can improve bone density, balance, coordination, digestion and sleep, and is associated with a longer lifespan. Why wouldn't you walk?

Jenn, a successful lawyer from Los Angeles, originally came in to see me to help her get through perimenopause. She had just turned 50 and noticed her clothes didn't fit anymore. When she finally weighed herself, she had gained 30 pounds. Along with the weight came fatigue, mood swings, trouble sleeping, and digestive issues. It's a tough place to be in, but Jenn's situation isn't unusual. As hormones fluctuate, the transition to menopause can be a bumpy ride, often lasting many years. However, exercise is one of the best remedies for the transition.

Since Jenn was sedentary and not used to exercising, I had her start by walking 20 minutes 5 - 7 days a week. I also introduced her to meal prepping. She started bringing her lunch to work instead of ordering takeout, which she ate daily for years. She didn't lose weight the first month, but Jenn didn't give up on herself. As soon as she got stronger and more energetic, we increased her walks to 30 minutes, then to 45 minutes almost daily. Walking worked well for her schedule. She kept a pair of walking shoes at work and walked on her lunch break. The weight started coming off, and a year later, Jenn not only lost all the weight, but she was sleeping better, got her energy back, no longer had intense mood swings, and resolved her digestive issues. All from the simple act of walking.

Most of us don't have to drive anywhere to walk, you could walk around the neighborhood where you live or work. If you live in an urban area, make a lunch date with a friend and walk to a restaurant or coffee shop. For most people a 20 minute brisk walk is about a mile. If you want to get the most out of walking then walk like you're late to a very important event. Walking fast gets the muscles pumping and blood flowing.

JOGGING / RUNNING

You probably don't need me to tell you that jogging and running are faster and more intense forms of walking. While the average walking pace is about 3 - 4 miles per hour, the average jogging pace is 4 - 6, and the average running pace is 6 or more miles per hour. Both jogging and running are great for your cardiovascular system and burn more calories than walking. A study from 2017 found runners live an average of 3 years longer than non-runners.[19] Running and jogging engage many muscle groups, can stimulate bone growth and

MOVE

improve density, and can boost your metabolism more than walking alone. The downside is they can be harder on the joints and lead to injury if you don't train properly. Be sure to start slow, warm up by walking for a few minutes, maintain proper running form to prevent injury, stay hydrated, and invest in good-fitting footwear. If you're new to running, I recommend getting a trainer or having someone observe your stride as you run to prevent injuries.

CYCLING

Cycling is another aerobic activity that's great for the heart, joints, muscles, bones, lungs, and immune system. It improves balance and coordination, builds endurance, reduces stress, anxiety, and depression and has been associated with better sleep.[20, 21]

Cycling is a great activity for those wanting to lose or manage their weight. The good news is it can be adapted to various fitness levels. If you're just starting out, make it fun by going on a low impact bike ride with your friends around town. If you're more advanced you can go on longer bike rides, go on bike friendly trails, take a spin class, or ride the bike at the gym. Just be sure when you're biking out on the town to stay in the bike lane, abide by the local traffic laws, and wear a helmet.

SWIMMING

If you like water, swimming can be one of the best workouts for you. It's a low impact, full body workout that gets the heart and lungs working while toning and strengthening your muscles.[22, 23] It's a great place to start if you have joint issues, back pain, or are recovering from an injury or surgery.

Swimming improves your motor skills by challenging your coordination and balance. It's one of those aerobic exercises that's suitable for all ages and fitness levels because it can be adapted to your individual needs. Make it social by joining a class or team, or make a day of it at the local pool.

RESISTANCE BANDS

Resistance bands are a low impact, joint friendly way to build strength and flexibility.[24] The lightweight bands are portable, compact, and cost effective making them ideal for home workouts. Resistance bands are very versatile, you can use them for a wide range of exercises that target all muscle groups for a relatively quick full body workout.[25] They come in different levels of resistance so you can adjust the intensity as needed.

The exercises done with resistance bands generally mimic the body's natural movements and are often used in physical therapy to help people gain strength, flexibility, balance, and stability. You can take a class at the gym, download an app, or watch youtube videos to learn how to use the bands.

YOGA

Yoga goes beyond the realm of exercise and deserves a book of its own. It's a blend of mind-body medicine, crossing over from movement to meditation to deep relaxation. Yoga uses the body to calm the mind through the breath, movements, postures, and stretches. It's one of those rare exercises that covers multiple areas of fitness making it ideal for those wanting to do cardio, flexibility, and balance exercises in one session.

Yoga as a physical medicine improves flexibility.[25] The more flexible you are the better your range of motion. Because yoga requires you to hold a pose while supporting your body weight, it can increase muscle strength, tone, balance, and stability.[26] People who do yoga regularly tend to have good posture and lower incidence of back and neck pain because they're more conscious of their alignment.

Yoga is also great for your cardiovascular system, improving the health of your heart, lowering blood pressure, and increasing circulation throughout the body.[26,27] Due to the focus on the breath, yoga is good for the lungs and improves oxygen delivery throughout the entire body. Yoga is associated with better sleep, immunity, digestion, mood, mental health and a lower occurrence of pain.[28,29] With all these benefits, why wouldn't you do yoga?

Keep in mind there are different kinds of yoga. If you're looking for a workout try hatha, vinyasa, ashtanga, or power yoga. If you're looking for relaxation try kundalini, restorative, or yin yoga. Be sure to read the class description before going so you don't end up in a class that only does chanting if you're looking for a workout.

RACKET SPORTS

Racket sports such as tennis, pickleball, squash, racquetball, badminton, and yes, even ping pong, are some of the best sports to play. According to a study published in the Mayo Clinic Proceedings, tennis players live on average 9.7 years longer than people who play other sports.[30] This is likely due to the fact that tennis and other racket sports are low-impact and less likely to cause injuries, they're social so they keep you connected with family and friends, and they're mentally stimulating which helps prevent cognitive decline and reduce the risk of dementia.

Playing racket sports can improve your cardiovascular health, help you maintain a healthy weight, improve bone health, and lower stress, anxiety, and depression.[31, 32] Many people like playing racket sports because of the social aspect. You can play with friends and family as well as make new, lifelong friends through the sport.

OVERCOME EXERCISE ANXIETY

Lao Tzu once said *the journey of a thousand miles begins with one step.* Starting anything new is terrifying, but the only way through fear is forward. I promise, once you're on the path, you'll realize it wasn't as hard as your mind was making it out to be. Instead of focusing on the end goal, focus on the process; one breath, one movement, one day at a time. There is only one step in front of you at the moment. Master that one before worrying about the next. Like all the other hard things you've done, you can do this too.

Make your workouts fun by bringing a friend along; you can go on a hike or bike ride together, swim at the local pool, or go out dancing if you like to dance. Buy yourself fun workout clothes and shoes and keep them somewhere obvious as a visual reminder. Make it a priority by putting it on your calendar. If all you have time for is a 20-minute walk, make it brisk. That'll get your blood flowing, and you'll feel so much better afterward.

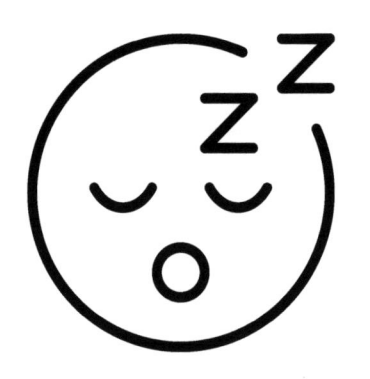

Sleep

I'm so good at sleeping that I can do it with my eyes closed.

~ Unknown

Sleep might be the strangest thing we do in the animal kingdom. After all, when we're sleeping, we're not doing anything that ensures our survival—eating, mating, tending to our young, building shelters, or fighting off predators. We're entirely useless for roughly eight hours, lying around in what appears to be a coma. So why do we sleep nearly one-third of our lives away?

It turns out sleep is as, if not more important than nutrition and exercise.[1] While nutrition and exercise build your body up, making you stronger and more resilient, restorative sleep repairs, fixes, and cleans so you're ready to go the next day. When you're sleeping well, you'll likely experience the following;

- Stronger immune system and reduced risk of disease.[2]

- Healthy weight.[3]
- Better skin health and overall appearance.[4]
- Increased metabolism.[5]
- Better sex drive.[6]
- Regulated blood sugar levels and appetite hormones.[5]
- Better digestion and healthier microbiome.[7]
- Lower blood pressure and better cardiovascular health.[8]
- Better memory and retention of new information.[9]
- Reduced anxiety and better moods.[10]
- Lower levels of inflammation.[11, 12]
- Decreased pain.[13]
- Lower risk of Alzheimer's and cognitive decline.[14, 15]

You can exercise and eat healthily all you want, but if you're not sleeping well, all that good work is going to waste. Bad sleep will win the battle every time. Poor sleep is associated with heart disease, diabetes, obesity, increased risk for infections, mood swings, irritability, anxiety, depression, poor memory, Alzheimer's, and even the big C word—cancer.[15, 16]

But before we scare ourselves into a frenzy over sleep, let me remind you that you won't wake up with cancer or Alzheimer's because you slept terribly last night. I know from experience being anxious about it doesn't help. So if you're having trouble sleeping, relax and take a few deep

SLEEP

breaths. Read through this chapter and implement some recommendations that resonate with you. Over time, you'll notice better sleeping patterns.

SLEEP-WAKE CYCLE

Internally speaking, there are two systems regulating the sleep-wake cycle. One is your circadian rhythm, the other is something called homeostatic sleep pressure. Most people have heard of circadian rhythm, it's your internal twenty-four hour clock nestled in a tiny area of your brain with a big name called the suprachiasmatic nuclei (SCN). It's what determines your rhythmic patterns of eating, drinking, sleeping, waking, urinating, moods, body temperature, metabolic rate, and hormone fluctuations.

The clock is strategically located where it can sense light and darkness entering the brain. When the sun starts going down, the SCN tells another area of the brain called the pineal gland, to release melatonin into the bloodstream. Melatonin is known as the hormone of darkness. It tells the body to get ready for bed. Once asleep, melatonin slowly decreases and as soon as light enters your eyes in the morning, the release of melatonin shuts off until the following evening. Interestingly, we all have slightly different circadian rhythms which explains why some of us are early birds while others are night owls.

The other system involved in sleep-wake cycles is called homeostatic sleep pressure. When you wake up, a chemical called adenosine starts building up in the brain creating chemical pressure. Adenosine is a byproduct of neurons using energy and acts as a sleep-inducing substance. The longer you're awake, the more the pressure builds, making you feel sleepier and sleepier until you finally fall asleep, generally 12-16 hours after waking. While you're sleeping, adenosine gets broken down and cleared from the body. This process slowly releases the pressure and encourages you to wake up. Ideally you feel awake and refreshed after a good night's sleep, then the cycle starts over again.

These two systems are not synchronized nor do they communicate with each other. However, many things interfere with them including electronic devices, caffeine, irregular sleep schedules, lack of exercise, stress, anxiety, environmental factors such as temperature and light, shift work, time changes, and jet lag.

STAGES OF SLEEP

Once we fall asleep, the brain cycles between two distinct stages throughout the night in 90 minute increments.[17] The first stage is non-rapid eye movement (NREM), and the other is rapid eye movement (REM).

During NREM sleep, the brain transitions from dozing off into a deep slumber. NREM sleep is characterized by slow brain waves and is when all the good stuff like cleaning, recovering, and recharging takes place. Think of it like when you're deep cleaning the house and moving furniture around

SLEEP

to sweep and vacuum the cobwebs and dust balls jammed into nooks and crannies. You kinda have to make a bigger mess before the house actually looks clean.

On the other hand, REM sleep is when dreaming takes place, emotions are processed, and memories move from short-term to long-term storage. It's characterized by faster brain wave activity similar to when we're awake. This is the stage where you put everything back in its proper place and tidy up. You really need both stages of sleep to complete the process.

The funny thing is, the balance between NREM and REM sleep isn't even throughout the night. The first half is dominated by NREM while the second half is dominated by REM. While many sleep experts emphasize NREM sleep, REM sleep is where a lot of the magic of memory consolidation and emotional processing happens. So if you're waking up early and can't get back to bed, you're missing out on a lot of valuable brain functions.

HOW TO SLEEP BETTER

Just like anything else, building good habits is the first step to establishing healthy sleep patterns. As you read through this section, take note of the recommendations that you think you're capable of doing and implement those first. Once those become habits, make additional changes until you are consistently sleeping well through the night. You'll know you're getting good sleep when you wake up feeling rested, are less reactive, and don't need caffeine to get your day started.

GET EARLY MORNING SUNLIGHT

A good night's rest starts in the morning. Believe it or not, early morning sunlight exposure is one of the primary predictors of how well you'll sleep in the evening. Our internal 24-hour clock synchronizes with the natural light-dark cycle of the environment. Morning light resets the system by telling the brain it's time to wake up. The blue morning light suppresses the production of melatonin, the hormone that tells the body it's time to sleep. It stimulates the production of serotonin, the happy chemical associated with better moods, and cortisol, the hormone that promotes wakefulness, increases energy, alertness, and cognitive function. Below are ways to get morning sunshine;

- **Go outside:** Aim for 5 - 10 minutes of direct morning sunlight exposure, within the first hour of waking. If it's cloudy or overcast, aim for 10 - 20 minutes. The light has to hit your eyes because that's how the SCN senses light and darkness. However, you can have your eyes closed while facing the sun because the light will penetrate through your eyelids. You also don't have to be staring directly at the sun as long as light is coming in through those photoreceptors. Windows block certain wavelengths of light so it's best to be outside to receive the benefits of full spectrum sunlight.

SLEEP

- **Take outdoor breaks:** Take your work breaks outside and pull up your sleeves to help with vitamin D synthesis. Even on cloudy days your sleep, mood, and mental state will benefit from the natural light, change of scenery, and fresh air.

- **Sit near a window:** If you can't get outside, then sit near a window. While you're not getting the full spectrum of light, natural light exposure helps synchronize your sleep-wake cycles and can enhance your overall mood.

- **Consider light therapy:** If you can't get outside nor be by a window, consider using light therapy devices that stimulate natural light. Tabletop ones can be placed on your desk, or you can replace overhead light bulbs with full spectrum bulbs and lighting.

LIMIT CAFFEINE INTAKE

A cup of Joe in the morning is an American ritual for a reason —it tastes great, can lift your mood, makes you more alert, and increases focus. The problem with caffeine is it competes with adenosine, the sleepy chemical in the brain, masking the build up of sleep pressure.[18] While the benefits of caffeine are coveted by anyone wanting to be alert and more productive, it can take up to 12 hours to completely clear your system. This means if you have a latte at noon, the caffeine can block your body's ability to recognize the build up of sleep pressure until midnight. The consequence is trouble falling and staying asleep. When we don't sleep well, we get tired, moody and have trouble focusing, leading to needing that caffeine high the next morning in order to be productive. But don't worry, you can still have your caffeine, just follow some recommendations to prevent sleep issues.

- **Time your caffeine:** When it comes to caffeine, dose and timing make the poison. Avoid all forms of caffeine including tea, soda, coffee, and chocolate 6 - 8 hours or more before you go to bed. I realize there are people out there who can have an espresso after dinner and have no trouble sleeping. But if you're like me and sensitive to the effects of caffeine, then stop your caffeine consumption early or don't indulge at all.

- **Opt for decaf:** If you can't give up your morning ritual, decaf is a great option. Note decaf doesn't mean no caffeine, so the same rules still apply. An 8 oz cup of regular coffee contains around 70 - 140 mg of caffeine, while an 8 oz cup of decaf can range from 2 - 7 mg of caffeine. So depending on how sensitive you are you might be able to get away with a cup of decaf in the afternoon. Just be honest with yourself, if it's interfering with your sleep, then substitute with an herbal caffeine free coffee substitute.

- **Watch your portion sizes:** Most people can tolerate a cup of regular coffee in the morning without it interfering with their sleep. But you're walking the line once you start getting into the 3 or more cups of coffee territory. Again, be honest with yourself, if it bothers you then scale back or switch to a caffeine free alternative.

- **Read labels:** You'd be surprised how many supplements, medications, sodas, coffee flavored desserts, protein bars, and energy drinks contain caffeine. Always check the labels and look up ingredients ahead of time to avoid overconsumption.

AVOID ALCOHOL

This is never a popular recommendation but research supports avoiding alcohol especially if you have trouble sleeping.[19] While many people have a glass of wine to help them relax and fall asleep, it actually interferes with the quality of sleep, leading to frequent awakenings, fragmented sleep, and reduced overall sleep duration.[20]

Alcohol reduces the time spent in REM sleep, which if you remember from above, is associated with vivid dreaming, memory, emotions, and cognitive function. This is why you feel slower and more sensitive the day after drinking. Another thing alcohol does is relax the muscles in the throat and airway contributing to sleep disorders like snoring and sleep apnea. Snoring interferes with both your's and your partner's sleep. Alcohol is a diuretic which means you'll likely be waking up multiple times in the night to pee. It can also disrupt blood sugar levels, one of the most common reasons for waking up in the middle of the night.

However, just like caffeine, dose and timing make the poison here. If you do choose to drink (which I am in no way advocating for because of all the other ill effects it has on the body), there are a few ways you can minimize (but not entirely eliminate) the effects it has on sleep;

- **Stop drinking a few hours before bedtime:** It takes hours for the liver to metabolize and break down alcohol. If you drink late at night then your liver will be trying to break down alcohol while you sleep. You'll end up waking up and have a hard time falling back asleep. If you choose to drink, do it early in the day.

- **Stick to one drink:** Higher alcohol consumption is associated with disrupted sleep. The more alcohol you consume, the longer it takes to metabolize and get cleared from the body.

- **Stay hydrated:** Alcohol is dehydrating so side effects such as dry eyes and mouth can cause discomfort and keep you up. The one-to-one ratio is a good rule to follow which is for every alcoholic drink, consume one 8 oz glass of water in between. It's also recommended to drink water before you go to bed and the next morning to rehydrate.

TIME YOUR MEALS & EAT FOR SLEEP

When I was in acupuncture college, I took classes at night so I could work during the day. Sometimes I wouldn't get home until 10 pm. I remember having difficulty falling asleep and couldn't figure out why. I told my herb professor about my sleeping problems, and he asked about my eating habits. I told him I ate dinner after getting home from class. He sternly said, "don't eat when you get home." I argued and told him I had to because I was hungry. He laughed and said, "then the patient doesn't want to get better."

Our body takes environmental cues for when it's time to sleep from three primary sources—light, temperature, and when we eat. Regular meal timing helps our internal 24-hour clock align with healthy sleep-wake cycles. If we eat late at night, our body thinks it's daytime, which keeps us awake by suppressing sleep signals. Eating late at night also interferes with sleep because the body has to digest lying down, making it difficult for food to move through the digestive tract. Nighttime eating can lead to indigestion, acid reflux, and even sleep apnea, all of which make it difficult to sleep.

The type of food you eat also plays a role in how well you sleep. For example, spicy foods can cause heartburn and indigestion, which are best avoided later in the day. Fatty foods take longer to digest and interfere with sleep due to discomfort. Sugary foods cause fluctuations in blood sugar, which can cause frequent waking at night.

However, many foods contain nutrients that support sleep. Poultry, dairy, nuts, and seeds contain tryptophan, an amino acid that produces hormones that help with sleep. Dark green leafy vegetables, nuts, seeds, legumes, and whole grains are high in magnesium, which promotes relaxation. Oatmeal and sweet potatoes are good sources of complex carbohydrates, are involved in the production of serotonin, and help with sleep. Eating these foods for dinner could help promote a good night's rest. The following is a list of foods that help with sleep;

BEING WELL

Food	Nutrient	Benefit
Nuts & Seeds (almonds, cashews, Brazil nuts, pistachios, walnuts, pumpkin, flax, chia, sesame, sunflower)	Magnesium, tryptophan	Promotes sleep, reduces stress
Bananas	Potassium, tryptophan	Regulates sleep-wake cycle, promotes sleep
Oats	Complex carbohydrates, magnesium, tryptophan	Promotes sleep, improves mood
Fatty fish (salmon, mackerel, sardines)	Omega-3 fatty acids	Improves sleep quality, reduces inflammation
Camomile tea	Apigenin	Promotes sleep, reduces anxiety
Tart cherries, pineapple	Melatonin	Promotes sleep, reduces inflammation
Kiwi	Vitamin C, serotonin, magnesium	Promotes sleep, reduces stress
Dark chocolate	Magnesium, tryptophan	Promotes sleep, reduces stress
Poultry (turkey, chicken)	Tryptophan	Promotes sleep, reduces stress
Dairy (milk, yogurt)	Calcium, tryptophan	Promotes sleep, reduces stress
Leafy greens (spinach, kale, Swiss chard, romaine)	Magnesium	Promotes relaxation
Legumes (lentils, chickpeas, black beans, edamame)	Tryptophan, magnesium, complex carbohydrates, fiber	Promotes sleep

SLEEP

Below are some guidelines to support better sleep using food;

- **Eat most of your calories early:** Have your larger meals earlier and the smallest meal for dinner. Eating this way helps keep your energy up during the day and allows for easy digestion and better sleep at night. As the saying goes, Eat breakfast like a king, lunch like a prince, and dinner like a pauper.

- **Choose sleep supporting ingredients:** Create dinner recipes containing sleep-supporting foods and nutrients while avoiding heavy and spicy foods interfering with digestion.

- **Have an early dinner:** Stop eating three hours before your usual bedtime. If you usually go to bed at 9 pm, finish your dinner by 6 pm. The only caveat here is if you tend towards low blood sugar, then have a small snack with complex carbs, protein, and fat to provide a steady release of energy and prevent blood sugar issues from waking you up at night.

- **Drink camomile tea:** Have a cup of camomile tea after dinner to promote relaxation.

MOVE YOUR BODY

It should be no surprise that exercise improves sleep. Humans are built to move. Exercise burns off extra energy, can lower anxiety and stress levels, reinforces the sleep-wake cycle, and improves sleep quality.[21] There's not much to it here. Move your body but don't do anything too vigorous close to bedtime.

- **Do what you like:** The best form of exercise is whatever you're willing to do consistently. Walking, running, hiking, swimming, cycling, dancing, strength training, yoga, you name it, have all been shown to have positive effects on sleep. The key is you want to do something everyday for at least 20 minutes.

- **Do it early:** The best time to exercise is in the morning because it increases mental alertness and raises body temperature. For these very reasons it's not recommended to exercise in the evening. As you get closer to bedtime you want your mind to relax and your body temperature to cool down. Aim to finish exercising a few hours before bedtime to give your body time to recover and cool down.

CREATE SLEEP RITUALS

Parents know the best way to get young kids to sleep is by having a consistent bedtime routine—dinner, warm bath, get into jammies, read bedtime stories, sing songs, put on soft music, kiss them, then turn off the lights and hope for the best. Any deviation from this routine and they turn into nocturnal monsters. The same is true for adults. We need time to transition from being busy and active to calm and asleep. The best way to do this is with sleep rituals.

SLEEP

Sleep rituals are activities you do every night to help you fall asleep. They help cue the body that it's time for sleep and can reduce stress and anxiety by allowing you to unwind. Examples of sleep rituals include;

- **Sipping on warm camomile tea in your favorite mug:** This soothing ritual helps you unwind by utilizing the compounds in camomile that help you relax.

- **Taking a warm bath:** Warm water helps your muscles relax and reduces anxiety and stress. Adding Epsom salt and lavender essential oil to the bath water can help lower cortisol, promote relaxation, and help you fall asleep faster.

- **Dimming all the lights in the house:** This promotes the production of melatonin and signals to your brain that it's time to wind down.

- **Turning on soft music:** Relaxing music calms the nervous system and quiets the mind.

- **Reading a book**: Reading helps divert your attention from the day's stress by getting lost in a good story.

- **Breathing exercises:** Breathing exercises help calm down your nervous system and shut down cortisol production.

- **Gentle stretches or restorative yoga:** Slow stretching or restorative yoga release tension in the body and promote relaxation.

BEING WELL

- **Good bedtime habits:** Habits like brushing your teeth, washing your face, and changing into comfortable jammies signal to your brain that it's time to go to bed soon.

BLISS OUT YOUR BEDROOM

Your bedroom should be a calming environment only used for sleep and intimacy. The brain is really good at making associations, so don't use your bedroom for entertainment, work, eating, or anything else distracting. If you do, it won't make the connection when you lay down that it's time to sleep. Your bedroom should be comfortable, cozy, cool, dark, clean, quiet, and free from clutter and electronics. Below are ways to make your bedroom a peaceful retreat;

- **Keep it cool:** I'll go into more detail in the next section, but generally, the ideal sleep temperature is around 20 C or 68 F.[22]

- **Invest in blackout curtains:** Any light can dampen the production of melatonin, that hormone that tells your body it's time to sleep. Blackout curtains block virtually all external light from entering the bedroom, creating a dark and friendly sleep environment. If light somehow sneaks in, consider wearing an eye mask for optimal sleep.

- **Keep it clean & clutter-free:** Clutter is distracting and can lead to feelings of stress and anxiety. Tidy spaces

SLEEP

promote a calm and peaceful atmosphere, making it easy to unwind.

- **Turn down the volume:** Noise can disrupt sleep. Create a peaceful ambiance with calming music, white noise, or quietness.

- **Comfortable bedding:** Your bed should be your most comfortable piece of furniture. Invest in the best pillows, sheets, mattresses, blankets, and duvets you can afford. Make sure you choose materials that are lightweight, breathable, and cozy to the touch. Weighted blankets have been shown to help people fall and stay asleep. They're like a constant hug and can calm the nervous system.

- **Electronics-free zone:** We have many opportunities to look at our devices during the day. Chances are, by the time you're ready for bed, you've already seen everything you needed to. So keep your phones, iPads, TVs, and other devices out of the bedroom. If you MUST bring in your phone, turn it off to resist the temptation of looking at it. The blue lighting on the screen shuts off melatonin production, confusing your body's circadian rhythm.

- **Soften the lights:** Sleep-supporting lighting is warm, soft, and dim. Invest in dimmer switches or adjustable lamps and warm-toned bulbs that resemble candlelight. Avoid bright or blue lights from screens. Cover up unnecessary lights from outlets and other bedroom devices with electrical tape.

BEING WELL

- **Make it smell nice:** The area of the brain associated with smell has a connection with brain regions involved with memory and emotions. This is why certain scents bring back happy memories. Scents can also influence neurotransmitter and hormone activity. Lavender enhances the activity of gamma-aminobutyric acid (GABA), a neurotransmitter that has a calming and soothing effect while reducing stress hormones such as cortisol. Experiment with calming scents such as lavender, chamomile, or jasmine to support a relaxing atmosphere in your bedroom.

- **Turn off WiFi:** WiFi emits low levels of electromagnetic radiation that some people are sensitive to. If this is you, turning it off while you sleep can reduce exposure and help you sleep better. It also limits potential distractions from devices since you won't be able to connect.

COOL IT DOWN

Have you ever tried falling asleep on a warm night without the help of air conditioning? It's not easy, right? That's because when it comes to sleep, our bodies prefer the environment to be on the chilly side, somewhere between 20 C or 68 F.[22]

Part of the reason for this is as we get ready to sleep, the body naturally starts to cool down, indirectly supporting the release of melatonin. If the room is too warm then the body's natural circadian rhythm gets thrown off, interfering with the signal that it's time to sleep.

Higher room temperatures also make it physically uncomfortable to sleep. It's not uncommon to wake up on hot nights due to an increase in heart rate, sweat, dehydration, restlessness, and even nightmares. Below are some ways to stay cool on warm nights;

- **Adjust the Thermostat:** Keep the temperature of your room around 20 C or 68 F. Start there and experiment to find the best sleeping temperature for you.

- **Warm Bath Before Bed:** Although this sounds counterintuitive, it actually promotes better sleep due to the drop in body temperature that occurs after the bath. The decrease in core temperature indirectly stimulates the release of melatonin, helping your body prepare for sleep.

- **Bedding:** Choose bedding that is lightweight and breathable like cotton and linen. Both these fabrics can keep you cool by promoting the flow of air and dissipating heat. Avoid synthetic materials as they can actually trap heat.

- **Cooling Accessories:** You can get pillows, mattress toppers and pads filled with cooling gel to regulate body temperatures and better disperse heat.

- **Cool Jammies:** Make sure your PJs are made from lightweight and breathable materials like cotton, linen, or bamboo. Like bedding, avoid synthetic fabrics because they trap heat.

BEING WELL

- **Stay Hydrated:** Dehydration can make you feel warmer. Make sure you're drinking enough liquids to stay hydrated without having to use the restroom during the night.

MIND YOUR SCREEN TIME

Let's be honest. How many times have you put on your favorite TV show and then proceeded to scroll Instagram on your phone the entire time your show was on? Don't be embarrassed; I'm guilty of this too. I love technology and being able to do anything I want from the comfort of my couch. It's pretty amazing, but it also has some equally amazing downsides. Having access to whatever I want at all hours of the day is a significant distraction. I now have to work harder to focus and be mindful of putting my device away when necessary.

But technology isn't going away—it will continue to weave its way into more and more areas of our lives. The key is to learn how to live without it harming our well-being. Like anything else, we have to build good habits around our devices. One way to change a habit is to replace it with a healthy one of equal or greater value.

For example, it's recommended to shut off all devices an hour before bedtime because they interfere with your circadian rhythm. Screens emit blue light, suppressing melatonin so your body doesn't get the signal that it's time to sleep. Devices also increase brain activity and stress,

SLEEP

especially when watching the news or engaging on social media, making it hard to fall asleep. Instead of being on your device, you could;

- Engage in a hobby like painting, drawing, or playing an instrument.
- Read a book.
- Journal.
- Listen to music, a podcast, or an audiobook.
- Connect with loved ones by playing games, cards, building a puzzle, or just hanging out.
- Call a friend you haven't spoken to in a while.
- Take a relaxing bath.
- Meditate or do restorative yoga.

The goal is to find something you like that's relaxing and doesn't interfere with your sleep-wake cycle. Try a few things out and give them time to stick. Over time you'll get used to your new routine and won't even miss your device.

GET IT OFF YOUR CHEST

Going to bed with a head full of thoughts is a sure way to guarantee you're not getting any sleep. You'll likely stay up, attempting to solve unsolvable problems that can't be addressed until the next day anyway. Writing down your thoughts and worries beforehand is an excellent way to counteract this.

Journaling is a form of self-expression and helps you externalize what's stuck in your head. By transferring your thoughts from your mind to paper, you can see them more objectively, creating distance and perspective. Journaling is therapeutic; it helps you express and process your emotions freely, gain insight, problem-solve, let go, and find closure on things that could otherwise keep you up for hours.

Grab some paper and start writing down everything on your mind. Separate them into categories of what can be done right away before you go to bed, and what needs to wait until tomorrow. If you are anxious, is it about something real and tangible, or is it hypothetical? Can it be dealt with right away, or can it wait until tomorrow?

Once you get everything off your mind, ending your journaling session with everything that went well is good practice. Journaling helps you shift your focus towards the positive and can help you cultivate a mindset of appreciation and gratitude, both conducive to a good night's rest.

SYNC YOUR SLUMBER

Once you're sleeping well, getting on a sleep schedule is going to help you establish healthier sleep patterns in the long run.[23] The body likes routines. A regular sleep schedule enhances how well and how long you sleep. It can also influence hormones like melatonin, which tell the body it's time to get ready to sleep. Everyone's sleep schedule is going to be slightly different but a good rule of thumb is set aside 8 hours for sleep, and your wake up time is more important than your bedtime. So if you usually need to be up by 6:00am, then get to bed by 10:00pm. Your sleep schedule could look something like this;

- **Early birds:** Bedtime 10:00pm; Wake-time: 6:00am.
- **Traditional 9-to-5ers:** Bedtime 11:00pm; Wake-time: 7:00am.
- **Night owls:** Bedtime: Midnight; Wake-time: 8:00am.

Remember that if you're having trouble sleeping then it's best to stay up until you actually feel tired. Don't try to go to sleep if you're not sleepy, this will make it harder to fall asleep. Once you start getting sleep, then you can get on a more regular sleep schedule.

GET OUT OF BED

There's nothing worse than waking up in the middle of the night and not being able to fall back to sleep. You anxiously lay there, watching the hours go by, hoping to fall back asleep. It's maddening.

Getting out of bed may sound counterintuitive, but it is one of the best things you can do in this situation. Lying awake in bed leads to conditioned arousal, where the brain starts associating the bed with being awake.

BEING WELL

Getting up prevents this association from taking place. Getting out of bed will also help to build up sleep pressure, so when you finally do jump back in bed, it's easier to fall asleep.

If you're up for 20 minutes or more, get out of bed, keep the lights dim, and do something calming. Stay off your screen, as the blue light is stimulating and will keep you from falling back asleep. Below are a few calming activities that can help you fall back asleep;

- **Brain dump:** Write everything down that's on your mind. Transferring thoughts to paper is a release and helps calm the mind. If you need to do anything, remind yourself there's little you can do in the middle of the night and that you'll take care of it in the morning.

- **Read a book:** Reading in dim light is relaxing and can help you fall back to sleep. Make sure whatever you read isn't stimulating. You don't want to read anything that's going to get you revved up. Choose light hearted stories or fiction that puts you back to sleep.

- **Meditate:** Meditation helps calm both the mind and body. We'll go over this in the next section but look for yoga nidra, body scans, or guided sleep meditations.

- **Breathing Exercises:** Certain breathing exercises promote relaxation and reduce stress. One good one you can do is box breathing, where you inhale for a count of four, hold for a count of four, exhale for a count of four, and hold for a count of four.

SLEEP

- **Listen to soothing music:** The right music can be very relaxing. You don't want anything with sudden volume or tempo changes. Try ambient, nature sounds, binaural beats, soft chants, or instrumental music.
- **Stretch or do yoga:** Yoga and stretching help to release stress and tension in the body. Try child's pose, legs-up-the-wall pose, or supportive bridge pose.

Remind yourself this is temporary, and you won't stay up forever. At some point you'll eventually fall asleep.

MEDITATE

One of the things that got me out of a bout with insomnia was meditation. I owe my life to it. It saved me from falling deeper into a pit of illness and pulled me up further than I thought was possible. Meditation is magic but in no way voodoo hoodoo. It's an ancient technique that teaches you how to stop the monkey chatter in your head. That's it. New meditators tend to make a bigger deal out of it than it is. When I first started meditating, I kept waiting for something to happen. At some point, fireworks would go off, and I'd suddenly be enlightened. That never happened, but I did learn to calm my mind and get clarity on what I wanted, including sleeping through the night again. Meditation reduces stress, helps you fall asleep faster, improves sleep quality, enhances the mind-body connection, and promotes relaxation and better emotional regulation.[24] Here are a few ways to practice meditation for better sleep;

- **Download a meditation app:** Using an app, especially when you're learning to meditate, can make meditation easy and take away a lot of the pressure of finding the right one and doing it right. Look for guided meditations for sleep, yoga nidra, non-sleep deep rest (NSDR), mantras for sleep, and body scan meditations. Some good meditation apps include WakingUp, which has yoga nidra and meditations for sleep, Headspace, Calm, and Insight Timer.

- **Make it a habit:** A consistent meditation practice can improve your brain. The more you do it, the better you'll get at calming your mind. Start small with short meditations and increase the duration and quantity over time. Even one minute a day can get you on your way to creating a regular meditation practice for better sleep.

- **Do guided meditation:** During guided meditation, a soothing voice, accompanied by calming music, guides you through a practice that redirects your attention away from racing thoughts so you can fall asleep. Guided meditations for sleep usually incorporate mindfulness techniques that have you focus on something, usually your breath, to bring your attention to the present moment. Focusing on your breath makes paying attention to those racing thoughts hard. Yes, you'll likely break focus, but bring your attention back to your breath when you do. Over time this becomes easier and can help insomnia.

- **Try yoga nidra:** Yoga Nidra, also known as yoga sleep, is closer to meditation than yoga. It's a guided meditation

SLEEP

that's typically done lying down. It helps release physical, mental, and emotional tension by having you focus on different parts of the body and mentally relaxing them. It has been shown to calm the nervous system, relieve stress and anxiety, and promote sleep when done before bed. You can even do it when you wake up in the middle of the night to help you fall back asleep. You can find scripts on youtube, but I'll also provide some in the guided meditation section on my website. Scan the QR code in the Resource section in the back of the book to be taken to the guided meditations.

MAKE LOVE

The sleep inducing benefits of making love are underreported, so I'll give them a shoutout in the name of science. Making love and climaxing is a great way to unwind, release tension, and forget about the worries of your day. This is because orgasms trigger the release of many hormones that promote relaxation, relieve stress, and provide feelings of well-being. For example;

- **Endorphins:** These are natural painkillers known as feel-good hormones because they elevate your mood and counteract stress. They're released during arousal and reach their peak during orgasm. Endorphins are responsible for that euphoric feeling during climax, creating a sense of bliss, calmness, and contentment post-orgasm.

- **Oxytocin:** Better known as the hormone of love, oxytocin promotes intimacy, connection, emotional bonding, and trust between lovers. It helps relax the nervous system and inhibits activity in the amygdala, the brain area involved with anxiety and stress response. Oxytocin alleviates pain, making it easier to fall asleep.

- **Prolactin:** Prolactin gets released after an orgasm to promote rest and recovery. It's also released during periods of deep relaxation and sleep and influences the duration and timing of sleep. Prolactin has analgesic properties and relieves pain.

- **Melatonin:** Orgasms enhance melatonin release, which tells your body it's time to sleep. During arousal and orgasm, various physiological processes, such as the relaxation response, the release of oxytocin, the increase in endorphins, and the release of prolactin after orgasm, all play a role in the production of melatonin, thereby contributing to better sleep.

- **Serotonin:** The "happy hormone" is associated with better moods, emotional connection, pleasure, sexual arousal, orgasm, and post-orgasmic relaxation. It's a precursor to melatonin, balances the sleep-wake cycle, calms the mind, relieves pain, and improves sleep.

The good news is that it doesn't matter how you arrive—even if you don't have a partner, having an orgasm can help you sleep better. However, some research shows that having a partner amplifies those sleep benefits.[25]

SLEEP

DON'T SNACK ON SLEEP

Naps are like little snacks of sleep. They're delicious, can give you energy, improve your mood, and even normalize your blood pressure. But napping also has a downside if indulged in for too long or too late in the afternoon.

The problem with napping is that it releases some of that healthy sleep pressure we've been building up during the day. Without enough sleep pressure, it will be harder to fall asleep when it's time for bed. Keep your naps short to minimize the amount of sleep pressure that gets released.

If you remember what I said a few pages back about the stages of sleep, the cycle between NREM and REM is about 90 minutes. Each stage of sleep gets progressively deeper until the cycle starts all over again. If you take a 40 minute nap, you might wake up in the middle of deep sleep, which isn't a natural place to wake up in the sleep cycle. When we wake up in deep sleep, we feel groggy, maybe even a little slow and confused. This is referred to as a sleep hangover, and it can take a full hour before you feel like yourself again.

Also people who have insomnia or trouble sleeping really need to get their nighttime sleeping in order before taking naps during the day. You want to build up as much of that sleep pressure as possible to help you fall asleep at night. Once you've established a healthy sleep pattern, you can start taking daytime naps. Below are my recommendations for napping;

- **20 minutes or less:** Too much napping can cause a sleep hangover when you wake up.

BEING WELL

- **No naps after 3 pm:** Napping past 3 pm is like snacking before a meal. It ruins your appetite for sleep.

- **No naps if you have insomnia:** Teach your body to sleep at night before you take daytime naps.

RESTFUL REMEDIES

Supplements are good options when you need an occasional nudge to help with sleep. They're great when you're traveling, have to deviate from your sleep schedule, or are more stressed than usual and need a good night's sleep. However, supplements shouldn't be relied on as a daily sleep aid since they're habit forming and can lead to dependency. The goal is to teach your body how to sleep on its own without the need for supplements or medication. That being said, below are some safe options that have less risk for dependency.

- **Valerian root** is an herb that contains compounds that have sedative effects. It's believed to modulate serotonin levels in the brain, relax muscles, and increase the activity of GABA, a neurotransmitter that calms the nervous system.[26]

- **Passion Flower** is an herb that helps calm the mind. It reduces nighttime awakenings, leading to more restful sleep.[27] It's also a good choice for those with menopausal-related sleep disturbances, as it may help keep the body cool.

SLEEP

- **Magnesium** is an essential mineral that many of us have low levels of.[28] It promotes relaxation, relieves muscle tension, and can calm an anxious mind. Magnesium comes in different forms, the best ones for sleep include magnesium glycinate or bisglycinate, as they are easily absorbed by the body. Magnesium threonate is another good one and may help to improve sleep by increasing chemicals in the brain that promote relaxation and sleep.

- **Camomile** is an herb used to promote relaxation.[29] It's high in the antioxidant apigenin, which binds to specific receptors in the brain that decrease anxiety and improve sleep.

- **Lavender oil** applied externally or diffused in the air is a soothing aroma that can improve sleep, reduce anxiety, and increase slow-wave sleep patterns associated with deep and restorative sleep phases.[30]

- **L-Theanine** is an amino acid found in green tea. It has a calming effect, helps reduce stress, and improves sleep.[31]

While sleep really does make an impact on our health, it's important not to get anxious or stressed when we're not sleeping well. Implement some of the above recommendations and take it one night at a time. You will eventually fall asleep.

Relax

Chronic stress is the ultimate junk food.

~ Herbert Herzog

Chronic stress is what got me into trouble so many years ago, and to be honest, if I'm not careful, it still does. Recently, a very good friend of mine critiqued my habits. She said the way I manage stress is by adding more stress.

Although I was annoyed with her uninvited insight, she was right. I tend to pile more and more on my plate until it breaks. But because this is my weak spot, it's also where I shine. I, more than anyone, know how to pivot the pendulum before it crashes, and I can also show you how. Not that you want to jump on my merry-go-round, but I can show you how to live a more balanced life while keeping up with the rigors of modern life.

BEING WELL

THE MODERN CAVEMAN'S DILEMMA

A common imagery in the world of stress science is the lion and caveman. The caveman is enjoying his day, probably relaxing in the sun with his cavewoman and cave babies, when suddenly a lion comes out of nowhere and tries to eat them.

A good stress response would be to run or stay and fight. Either way, the stressed caveman's adrenal glands would release cortisol and adrenaline, stress hormones that prep the body for what's about to go down. The nervous system would send all the blood and energy to the muscles and increase the breathing rate so he could run faster or fight harder. Other organs would temporarily shut down so he wouldn't be bothered by digesting or needing to find a bathroom while saving his family.

Assuming our ancestors won, everything would go back to normal. Blood would return to organs, the adrenal glands would stop releasing stress chemicals, and breathing and heart rates would normalize. The entire family would go back to sunbathing on a rock.

This is how our bodies were designed to deal with stress; in short bursts. We'd deal with a significant stressor for 30 minutes, then go back to napping under a tree or whatever cave people did for fun.

Fast forward 10,000 years, and you'll find a different setup. Hustle and bustle is the modern person's motto—do more, create more, work more, eat more, drink more, worry more, exercise less, relax less, and sleep less. There's no

RELAX

napping under a tree unless it's scheduled on your calendar, which you probably double booked yourself at that time anyway. We're constantly stressed and under pressure to perform, and it rarely lets up.

The problem here is that our ancient bodies haven't caught up with modern living. Our nervous systems still deal with stress like the caveman's did—by releasing chemicals, pumping blood and energy to muscles, and shutting down digestion and other organs. In 30-minute increments, all is well, but in the long term, we start to see a garden variety of disease kick in, directly linked to chronic stress.

Imagine if you were constantly battling a lion 24/7. It'd be exhausting. At some point, you'd break down and probably lose the battle. This happens when you set a deadline after deadline, work long hours, don't sleep, make terrible food choices, pull all-nighters, and drink caffeine and energy drinks all day to self-medicate and remedy the situation. You're stressing your body out. It does its best to keep up, but will eventually break down at this pace. Tag on a viral or bacterial infection, the death of a loved one, or the birth of a child and your body is toast.

Remember what I said above about blood being pumped away from vital organs during stress? This means they're not getting the nutrients they need to perform, repair, and rejuvenate themselves. On top of that, many of us are addicted to the adrenaline rush and dopamine that floods our brains when we're under pressure. They provide a heightened sense of alertness that gives us laser-sharp focus. But chronic stress depletes these very chemicals, leaving us burned out and exhausted overtime. It's no wonder many diseases are directly linked to chronic stress.[1, 2, 3]

Yet, here we are, living in the 21st century. Unless you can move to a mountaintop and hire someone to do everything for you, it's unrealistic to expect you to live without stress and responsibilities. They're not going away. The key is to recognize the source and how it's manifesting in your body, get rid of what you can, and practice healthy ways to unwind and mitigate the impacts of stress. Read on to find out how to do that.

GET FAMILIAR WITH YOUR TRIGGERS

The first step in stress management is identifying your triggers. What is it that's causing your symptoms? Common triggers come from workplace dynamics, job security or finances, your own or loved one's health concerns, family and relationship dynamics, concerns about safety and security, politics, technology, the news, social media, pressure related to academic performance, and environmental concerns. How can you pinpoint your root causes?

Start with self-reflection and journaling. Think back to the last time you didn't feel stressed, and then move forward in time from there. You can write down any changes, events, or situations that happened around the time you started feeling stressed. Maybe it had to do with your job, the birth of your baby, the death of a loved one, or the expectations and pressures you placed on yourself.

RELAX

You can also take a hard look at any lifestyle factors that can be contributing to the feelings of stress. Think caffeine, lack of exercise, poor sleep habits, excessive alcohol use, etc.

KNOW YOUR SYMPTOMS

Symptoms of stress manifest in different ways for different people. It usually breaks down your weakest link first. If you're someone with a bad stomach who seems to get every bug going around, then the symptoms of stress will likely show up in your gut. If you carry the world's weight on your shoulders, stress will likely show up in your neck, shoulders, and upper back. Weight gain will probably be your first symptom if you gain weight easily. If you're prone to anxiety, then you guessed it, you'll likely end up with more anxiety. Below are some symptoms of stress to look out for;

- **Pain:** Headaches and muscle tension, especially in the neck, shoulders, and back.

- **Digestion:** Nausea, diarrhea, constipation, cramps, appetite changes, weight gain or loss.

- **Sleep:** Difficulty falling and staying asleep, restlessness at night.

- **Immune:** Frequent colds or infections.

- **Cardiovascular:** Rapid heartbeat, chest pain.

- **Respiratory:** Rapid or trouble breathing.

BEING WELL

- **Emotional Signs:** Mood swings, short temper, anxiety, depression, restlessness, withdrawal, substance abuse, decreased libido, compulsive behaviors such as nail biting or pulling out hair.
- **Cognitive Signs:** Forgetfulness, difficulty making decisions, worry, pessimistic outlook.
- **Other:** Difficulty swallowing, dry mouth, fatigue.

This is just a shortlist. Stress can manifest in other ways and may not even be noticeable. It might manifest as a silent health condition, so it is important to get regular checkups. So what can you do about it?

BURN OFF STRESS

Remember what we said about stress raising cortisol and adrenaline and pumping blood to your muscles? You can burn off stress by exercising. Exercise also releases endorphins, those feel-good chemicals serving as an outlet for mood-related symptoms.

The best type of exercise will be whatever you like and are willing to do. Aerobic, strength training, sports, stretching, you name it, can help lower stress and increase those feel-good chemicals. Walking, running, jogging, cycling, swimming, dancing, lifting weights, stretching, hiking out in the sunshine, and playing sports with friends are all great ways to burn off stress.

RELAX

Yoga, tai chi, and qi gong incorporate mind/body movements, often called 'meditation in motion.' The whole point of yoga is to get your body to a place of relaxation so you can meditate. So try these out and find what works best for you. Consistency is key, so start where you are and increase your exercise over time.

RELAX HARDER

This may sound counterintuitive, but you have to put effort into relaxing. Simple things like slow, deep breathing or meditation can be challenging for someone with a racing mind. If done incorrectly can actually cause more stress rather than relieve it. However, every battery eventually dies unless it gets recharged. So, schedule relaxation into your calendar and commit to doing it. Below is a short list of various stress-relieving activities that many of my patients have found helpful;

- **Belly Breathing:** Deep breathing activates the body's relaxation response and is one of the best ways to calm the nervous system. When we're anxious or stressed, our breathing becomes rapid and shallow, limiting the amount of oxygen our body receives and the amount of carbon dioxide it releases. Intentionally taking slow and deep breaths can normalize respiration and calm an anxious mind. One of the easiest breathing exercise is called belly breathing where you breath deep into your belly and see it rise and fall. Try this:

- Place your hands on your belly.

- Breathe in through your nose for a count of four, being mindful to fill your belly.

- Hold it for a count of four.

- Exhale slowly through your mouth for a count of four.

- Pause for a count of four.

- Repeat several times until you feel your body and mind relaxing. You should feel your belly rise and fall with each breath.

- **Progressive Muscle Relaxation:** Progressive muscle relaxation (PMR) is a technique where you deliberately tense muscle groups and then relax them. It helps to relieve physical tension and leads to mental calmness. In each area of your body, you will tense the muscle groups for five seconds, then release and relax for five seconds before moving on to the next muscle group. If you have an injury, skip tensing the muscles in that area and move on to the next muscle group.

    - Find a comfortable place where you can lay down and won't be disturbed.

    - Close your eyes and take a few deep breaths in and out.

    - **Forehead:** Starting with the forehead, raise your eyebrows and hold for five seconds. Then relax for five seconds.

- **Eyes & Nose:** Close your eyes tightly and scrunch your nose.
- **Jaw:** Clench your jaw and bite down.
- **Neck:** Tilt your head back, stretching the front of your neck. You should feel the back of your neck tense up.
- **Shoulders:** Shrug your shoulders up to your ears.
- **Upper Limbs:** Clench your fists and tighten the muscles in your arms.
- **Chest:** Take a deep breath and hold it in.
- **Back:** Arch your back.
- **Abdomen:** Round your back and tighten the muscles on your abdomen
- **Buttocks:** Tighten your glutes.
- **Lower Limbs:** Point your toes and tighten your leg muscles.

- **Spend time in Nature:** The therapeutic benefits of nature have been the subject of many scientific studies. A scientific review found 92% of people who engaged in outdoor environments demonstrated consistent improvements across any health outcome.[4] Another review found an association between time spent out in nature and improved cognitive function, brain activity, blood pressure, mental health, and physical health.[5] People who spend time out in nature tend to be calmer and happier. Nature's sights, sounds, and smells stimulate the senses in a way that calms the nervous system. You can go for a walk around a park or botanical garden, a hike, a bike ride, the beach or a lake, etc. Whatever gets you out of the house or office and around greenery will do. Even sitting under a tree for as little as 10 - 15 minutes can improve your mood and leave you relaxed and rejuvenated.

- **Journal:** Journaling is a way to release pent-up emotions and calm the mind. Putting feelings into words can help you process stressful experiences and gain a fresh perspective. It's an effective way to develop coping mechanisms and constructively manage stress. Start by writing down what's causing your stress. It's ok if you don't know, the very process of writing may reveal your triggers. While journal entries don't need to be lengthy, regular and free-flowing writing can significantly reduce stress levels.

Depending on what you love, many other things can be relaxing. Reading, taking a warm bath, getting a massage, listening to music, doing yoga, playing with your pet, hanging out with friends, and just laughing are great ways to relax and can significantly affect your overall stress levels.

NOURISH YOUR NERVES

By now you probably know diet has a lot to do with our health, and stress management is no exception. The foods you eat can either exacerbate or calm down the stress response. Unhealthy foods cause inflammation, a slow-burning internal stress that eventually breaks down your body. On the other hand, a healthy, balanced diet with lots of nutrients gives you energy and will help your body deal with stress.

Many people 'stress eat' to make them feel better. The problem is they're not overeating on celery, lettuce, and carrots—they're overeating on ultra-processed foods loaded with simple sugars, refined oils, and salt. These foods are guaranteed to cause weight gain. This is why it's so important to avoid buying ultra-processed foods in the first place. It's much harder to stress-eat unhealthy foods if they're not in your house. Of course, you can go out and purchase them, but that extra step might save you from mindless eating.

Below is a list of healthy foods that help combat the physiological effects of stress. I'm sure you won't be surprised to see the list pretty much lines up with the healthy diet listed in the EAT chapter;

- **Complex Carbs:** Oatmeal, quinoa, and sweet potatoes stabilize blood sugar, boost serotonin, a feel-good neurotransmitter, and provide sustained energy.

- **Fatty Fish:** Wild caught salmon, mackerel, and sardines are rich in omega-3 fatty acids that reduce stress hormones and promote brain health.

- **Leafy Greens:** Spinach, kale, and Swiss chard contain magnesium, which can regulate cortisol and relax the nervous system.

- **Nuts & Seeds:** Almonds, walnuts, macadamia, pecans, chia, flax, and pumpkin seeds are all great sources of vitamins and minerals that can boost your resilience to stress.

- **Probiotic-Rich Foods:** Yogurt, kefir, sauerkraut, kimchi, and miso support the health of the gut, which in turn, helps brain health and stress response.

- **Citrus Fruits:** Oranges, grapefruits, and lemons are high in vitamin C, a nutrient that reduces stress and boosts the immune system.

- **Berries:** Strawberries, blueberries, raspberries, and blackberries contain antioxidants and vitamin C, nutrients that support your body's resilience to stress.

- **Dark Chocolate:** Contains antioxidants, polyphenols, and magnesium, all helpful in managing stress.

- **Avocados:** Rich in vitamin E, B vitamins and potassium, which support overall health and wellbeing.

- **Bananas:** Good source of vitamin B6 and mood-boosting carbohydrates.

- **Turkey & Tofu:** Both contain tryptophan, an amino acid that increases serotonin levels in the brain.

- **Seaweed:** Contains vitamins and minerals that support adrenal health and stress response.

- **Water:** Dehydration can raise cortisol levels and lead to signs and symptoms of stress.

RELAX

CHOOSE HEALTHIER VICES

Chronic stress leads to brain and body fatigue, which is why many of us crave coffee and sugar to get us through stressful times. The problem with stimulants like caffeine is that they draw on your adrenals to boost energy. They increase cortisol production, your body's primary stress hormone, which can cause anxiety, jitteriness, nervousness, and tension. In other words, stimulants cause more stress rather than relieve it. They also interfere with sleep, raise blood pressure, can cause overstimulation, and lead to dependency. The good news is there's plenty of healthy alternatives. Look for herbal teas, decaffeinated coffee, green smoothies, chicory root coffee, adaptogenic herbs like ashwagandha, rhodiola, eleuthero, schisandra, cordyceps, maca, gotu kola, and ginseng.

Another common vice people depend on to cope with stress is alcohol. Unfortunately, alcohol is a depressant. While it may seem like the answer to your problems, it's only masking them and preventing you from developing healthier coping mechanisms. Like stimulants, depressants cause mood swings and depression, interfere with sleep, and lead to health problems and dependency. Alternatives to alcohol include sparking water, mocktails, kombucha, golden milk, coconut water, and herbal teas made with calming herbs such as reishi mushroom, passionflower, valerian root, kava, camomile, skullcap, lemon balm, ashwagandha, and holy basil. You can drink your replacement beverage out of one of your nicer glasses so you can keep the ritual without the consequence.

GO PLAY

Do you remember how fun it was running around on the playground, sliding down slides, or swinging on the swings as a kid? When did we decide play was only for children? Maybe sliding down a bumpy slide isn't your thing anymore, but there are adult forms of play that can bring you the same amount of joy. Play is a necessary activity that boosts creativity, lowers stress hormones, lifts the spirits, and helps us connect with our inner child and loved ones.

A big problem I see is people are so wrapped in responsibilities that playtime has become a thing of the past. Most of us have forgotten how to play. But life isn't meant to be all work—humans are built to enjoy themselves and have fun. Ask yourself these questions;

- What does fun mean to me?
- What would I do if I had an entire day off with no obligations?
- What can I do to include more play in my life?

Fun may not look the same to you now as it did in the past. This is where exploring and trying new activities comes in handy. Maybe your idea of fun is going to the movies, having a spa day, going out to dinner or dancing, cooking, photography, playing cards, board games, or sports, coloring with your kids, painting, traveling, going to a concert, gardening, or playing video games. Whatever it is, remember that the essence of play lies in the joy it brings you. It's about being in the moment and having fun. So make time to do the things you love. Your inner child will thank you.

RELAX

GET YOUR ZZZZZS

Sleep is so important that I dedicated an entire chapter to it. Sleep and stress have a bidirectional relationship, meaning they influence each other. Stress can lead to poor sleep, and poor sleep can lead to stress.[6] This is why nurturing both areas is essential; neither gets knocked out of balance.

Chronic stress leads to increased cortisol, the stress hormone involved in wake response. Higher cortisol levels mean a more challenging time falling and staying asleep. Stress also reduces the amount of REM sleep you get, which is the critical phase of emotional regulation and memory formation.

Poor sleep can lead to trouble thinking, mood problems, hormonal imbalance, health issues like obesity, diabetes, cardiovascular disease, and lowered immunity.

Refer to the SLEEP chapter for ways to get better sleep.

LEAN ON FRIENDS

Humans are social creatures, and relationships are very important to us. Having a few close friends to lean on could make stressful situations bearable. They can pull you out of your head, make you laugh, and nudge you to relax and let go.

A good friend will listen to you when you're feeling overwhelmed, offer a fresh perspective, provide physical comfort, take over things on your to-do list, distract you from the stress, hold you accountable, and encourage you to move forward and seek help when needed.

People are usually more than willing to help, so don't be afraid to ask for help when needed.

UNPLUG

While it's important to stay up-to-date with current events, you don't need to wallow in them all hours of the day. Information overload is a real thing and can lead to cognitive fatigue, depression, anxiety, and increased stress.

While we tend to believe the news delivers balanced information, it is heavily biased toward the negative because negativity gets more views. However, continuous exposure to negative news leads to heightened stress and feelings of hopelessness and fear. People who constantly watch the news are on edge. One small thing could set them off and cause them to overreact. Below are ways to watch the news and engage with social media responsibly;

- **Limit Exposure:** Set specific times to check the news and social media during the day. Avoid endless doom scrolling.

- **Curate Content:** Only follow positive, educational accounts that bring you joy. Delete accounts that stress you out and bring up negative emotions. You don't need them.

RELAX

- **Digital Detox:** Take regular breaks from social media. If you check your accounts daily, try going 2 - 3 days without checking your accounts.

- **Fact-Check:** Make sure the news you're consuming is from reputable sources, and always fact-check to avoid the stress of misinformation.

You can donate money, show up to important events that are meaningful to you, and post something on social media about it, but when you're finished, let it go and do something else. World catastrophes are always happening. If you keep yourself knee-deep in them, they'll eventually pull you under.

MASTER YOUR TIME

There's nothing worse than putting something important off then having to rush and get it done last minute. The anxiety and stress that come with procrastination are not worth it. Having good time management skills and staying organized offers a sense of control and direction. Below are ways to manage your time and stay on track;

- **Prioritize Tasks:** Decide what needs to get done first.

- **Set specific goals:** Break them down into smaller tasks to make them more manageable.

- Use time management techniques:
  - **Pomodoro technique:** Work for 25 minutes, then take a 5 minute break.

135

- **Time blocking:** Dedicate specific blocks of time to particular tasks.
- **Two-minute rule:** If it will take less than two minutes—do it now.
- **Plan Ahead:** Use daily planners, and digital to-do lists to allocate tasks for specific days and times
- **Minimize Distractions:** Avoid being sidetracked by distractions. Close your office door, wear noise canceling headphones, and turn off social media and text messaging on your devices while you're trying to work.
- **Stay Organized:** Keep your workspace tidy so you don't have to rummage through to find your materials while working.

KINDLY DECLINE

Setting boundaries and saying no is a big part of stress management. If you commit yourself to something you don't want to do or know you can't get done in time, you will be stressed out, anxious, and resentful.

Declining kindly is a way of saying no without burning bridges. While initially it may feel uncomfortable to say no or set boundaries, you'll feel better in the long run. It involves being self-aware enough to know your limits, priorities, and values and consistently staying within your boundaries.

Saying no in a kind way involves empathy, tact, and clear communication so you can understand where the other person is coming from. It allows you to say no without being rude, vague, or misleading. Always express gratitude and appreciation for the offer or request and, when possible, offer alternatives like another person who can complete their request.

Fewer commitments mean more time for doing things you love and actually want to do, bringing balance to your life and lowering stress. A double win!

While stress is inevitable, it doesn't have to run your life. By recognizing your triggers, signs, and symptoms, you can take proactive steps to manage and alleviate its effects. The strategies discussed above are tools and gateways to a happier, more balanced life. By regularly practicing stress-relieving activities, you can cultivate a life rich in purpose and joy.

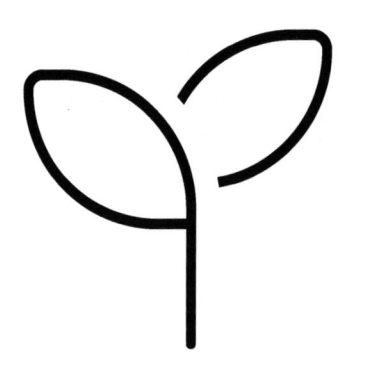

Detox

*The body is designed to detox naturally,
but sometimes it needs a little help.*

~ Dr. Andrew Weil

I consider myself cautiously optimistic and incredibly lucky to be living in modern times. Never before have we had so many resources available to us. We have cars and planes that take us all over the world, TVs and Playstations to entertain us, and iPhones that connect us to anything we've ever wanted whenever we want it. Freshly caught salmon is immediately flown across the world so water-lacking inlanders can indulge in fresh sushi. Hawaii exports mangos and papayas, so even people in northern latitudes can enjoy an abundance of tasty, sweet tropical fruits any day of the week. Most of us have access to the best technology, medical care, and education that previous generations could never even dream of.

Yet, every coin has two sides. The flip side of modern luxury is a world polluted with synthetic chemicals that are not only harming our health, but the entire planet. We live in the most toxic time in history, with thousands of new chemicals introduced yearly.

The United Nations Environment Programme (UNEP) has reported that industries have introduced over 350,000 synthetic chemicals since the industrial revolution, and only a small percentage of those have been tested for potential impacts on human health.[1] Many are 'forever chemicals,' meaning they take thousands of years to break down in the environment and build up in the tissues of living organisms like humans.[1] Below is a list of toxic substances and their impact on human health;

- **Pesticides:** Glyphosate, Organophosphate, Atrazine. Linked to cancer, Parkinson's, Alzheimer's, reproductive problems, respiratory issues, birth defects, immune dysfunction, and skin and eye irritation.[2, 3, 4]

- **Heavy Metals:** Lead, Mercury, Aluminum, Cadmium, Arsenic, and Bromines. Associated with cancer, neurological problems, kidney and heart issues, reproductive concerns, and skin and eye disorders.[5, 6, 7]

- **Plastics and Plastic Derivatives:** Bisphenol A (BPA), Phthalates, Polyvinyl Chloride (PVC), Microplastics, Styrene, Polycarbonate, PFAS, Flame Retardants, polychlorinated biphenyls (PCBs). Linked to reproductive, neurological, developmental, endocrine disorders, and cancer.[8, 9]

DETOX

- **Food Preservatives:** Sulfites, Nitrates, MSG, Sodium Benzoate, Propyl Gallate, Aspartame, BHT. Associated with cancer, allergic reactions, gastrointestinal and neurological problems, and developmental delays.[10, 11]

- **Artificial Sweeteners:** Aspartame, Acesulfame K, Equal, Neotame, Nutrasweet, Saccharin, Sucralose, Splenda, Sweet n' Low. Linked to metabolic issues like insulin resistance and type 2 diabetes, weight gain, cardiovascular conditions, digestive problems, and allergic reactions.[12, 13, 14, 15]

- **Cosmetic Chemicals:** Tar, DEA/TEA/MEA, Fragrance, Formaldehyde, Hydroquinone, Lead, Mercury, Mineral Oil, Oxybenzone, Parabens, Phthalates, PEG, Sodium Laurel Sulfate, Talc, Toluene, Triclosan. Associated with various health problems.[16, 17]

- **Refined Sugar:** Table sugar (sucrose), High Fructose Corn Syrup (HFCS), Brown Sugar, Powdered Sugar (Confectioner's Sugar), Cane Juice, Cane Syrup, Corn Syrup, Agave, Maltose, Dextrose, Fructose. Associated with weight gain, type 2 diabetes, heart disease, fatty liver, tooth decay, cancer, cognitive decline, poor nutritional habits, depression, accelerated skin aging.[18, 19, 20, 21]

- **Refined Vegetable Oils:** Soybean, Corn, Canola, Cottonseed, Sunflower, Safflower, Grapeseed, Palm, Peanut oils, and Margarine. Associated with inflammation and related disorders.[22]

The good news is that our bodies have an incredible built-in detoxification system that constantly filters harmful substances and removes them from the body. However, it wasn't designed to take on a chemical burden like this. Therefore, to stay healthy and avoid disease, you must proactively minimize exposure to toxins and do things that support your body's natural detoxification pathways.

This section is about supporting your body's natural detoxification system using specific lifestyle practices, nutrition, and supplements.

DETOX 101

The liver is by far my favorite organ. Not only is it in charge of breaking down everything we consume, but it runs your entire detoxification system, filtering blood and removing toxins, alcohol, drugs, and other harmful substances.[23] It makes bile, which helps remove toxic substances and aids in the digestion of fats. It metabolizes and breaks down hormones so they don't build up and cause hormone-related health issues.

The liver uses a two step process called biotransformation to break down substances. 'Bio' means life, and 'transformation' means change or alteration. In the first step, the liver uses vitamins C, E, and B vitamins and minerals like iron and magnesium to break down substances. This is why nutrition is essential for detoxification—nutrients fuel the process. The downside of step 1 is that the altered substance can become even more toxic. That's where antioxidants (our body's defenders) like Glutathione and vitamins C and E step in to protect us. Alcohol, certain medications, and environmental toxins interfere with this step, so avoid them when actively supporting your detoxification pathways.

Step 2 makes the toxins harmless and prepares them for excretion from the body. For this to happen, the liver needs Glutathione, B5, B6, folate, B12, magnesium, molybdenum, amino acids (building blocks of proteins) like glycine, taurine, glutamine, cysteine, and methionine. Foods rich in sulfur, like garlic and onions, and colorful fruits and veggies contain the nutrients the liver needs for both steps. However, you can supplement with nutraceuticals if you're not getting enough nutrients from your diet.

Once the liver processes toxins, they need a way to exit the body. The lymphatic, gastrointestinal, urinary, respiratory, and integumentary (skin) systems help eliminate waste products from the body. The lymphatic system is a star player of the immune system. Like a freeway, it shuttles waste and toxins out of the cells and brings them to holding stations called lymph nodes, where they get filtered and neutralized. The filtered fluid enters the bloodstream, is filtered again by the kidneys, and exits the body as urine. The gastrointestinal tract takes broken-down products from the liver and eliminates them with your bowel movements. The lungs eliminate gaseous waste like carbon dioxide and expel airborne toxins through exhalation. The skin can release some toxins and waste products through sweat, but not to the same extent as the urinary or gastrointestinal tract.

SIGNS YOU COULD USE DETOX SUPPORT

Think of your body like your house. Regular cleaning keeps it clean and smelling fresh, but what happens if you don't dust, organize, take out the trash, or do the dishes? Dust, garbage, and clutter accumulate, making your living environment chaotic and stinky.

Similarly, our bodies need regular cleaning. When any of the above systems are overwhelmed, toxins accumulate in adipose (fat) tissue, the brain, nervous system, and bones and cause various health problems.[24, 25, 26, 27] This process is called toxic overload and leads to symptoms like fatigue, headaches, dizziness, sugar or caffeine cravings, water retention, swollen eyes or face, nausea, vomiting, rashes, irritability, anxiety, depression, mood swings, weight gain, memory problems, difficulty concentrating, heart arrhythmias, bad breath, and body odor.

There are different levels of detoxing. Some require you to be under the care of a medical provider. However, what I recommend is gentle enough to be done on your own daily since it's sustainable and non-restrictive. Below, you'll find ways to support your body's natural detoxification process.

STOP PUTTING TOXINS IN YOUR BODY

The first step in assisting your body's natural detoxification system is to avoid toxins in the first place. Stop eating conventional food sprayed with pesticides, stop drinking

DETOX

alcohol, lower your intake of sugar and ultra-processed foods, invest in an air purifier and water filter, change out your personal care products and cleaning products for green ones, replace plastic containers and water bottles with glass or other non-toxic materials, and so on.

Be patient with yourself, as there's a steep learning curve. It took me an entire year to replace all my personal care and cleaning products with green ones and go plastic-free. Take your time, start with one thing on the list and work your way through the worksheets provided in the additional resource section near the end of the book.

FLUSH OUT YOUR BODY

Water isn't just about quenching thirst—it's one of the most potent yet underutilized remedies for better health. It should be the first place you start when looking to clean out your system. Every sip of water is like a mini cleanse, showering the inside of your body. As it goes through the entire body, it helps to dissolve and remove toxins through urine.[28] It also helps in the breakdown of food and absorption of nutrients in the digestive tract and prevents constipation. Like a plant perks up when watered, every cell thrives and works better when well-hydrated.

As mentioned earlier, to ensure your cells are hydrated, drink half your body weight in ounces throughout the day. Add electrolytes when working out, on hot days, or when you sweat more than usual.

BEING WELL

EAT DETOX FRIENDLY FOODS

Diet is one of the easiest and most natural ways to detox the body. Eat organic, nutrient-dense, whole foods and minimize your exposure to chemicals, ultra-processed foods, alcohol, and other toxins. You can eat various fruits and vegetables, especially those rich in antioxidants, vitamins, and minerals that support both phases of liver biotransformation. There are many great foods to choose from. Aim to eat a variety of foods from the list below throughout the week.

- **Cruciferous vegetables**, including broccoli, Brussels sprouts, cauliflower, cabbage, radish, bok choy, arugula, collard greens, watercress, and wasabi, contain compounds such as glucosinolates that support phase 1 and 2 of biotransformation and help break down and eliminate toxins from the body. They're high in antioxidants that protect the liver from damage, are high in fiber that supports bowel movements, and aid in eliminating toxins from the digestive tract.

- **Allium vegetables** such as garlic, onions, leeks, chives, green onion, and shallots are rich in sulfur-containing compounds such as allicin, which support phase 1 and 2 of biotransformation and protect the liver from damage caused by toxins. They're rich in antioxidants like quercetin and vitamin C, neutralizing free radicals and reducing oxidative stress. They stimulate glutathione production, reduce inflammation, and can support the immune system, supporting the liver's natural detoxification process.

- **Cilantro, or coriander** contains compounds that bind to toxic metals such as lead and mercury and usher them out of the body. It's high in several antioxidants that protect your cells from damage. Cilantro has anti-inflammatory properties and can stimulate digestive enzymes that help with digestion.

- **Green Tea** contains catechins, compounds that protect the liver from damage and improves the liver's ability to metabolize and eliminate toxins.

- **Turmeric** is high in curcumin, a potent anti-inflammatory compound that protects the liver and supports its ability to metabolize and eliminate toxins.

- **Artichokes** contain compounds called cynarins, which stimulate the production and release of bile that carries waste products of the liver. They're high in antioxidants that protect the liver from damage and high in fiber, supporting digestion and regular bowel movements. Artichokes promote liver regeneration and feed the healthy bacteria in your gut.

- **Berries** contain antioxidants like flavonoids, anthocyanins, and vitamin C, lowering inflammation and supporting overall liver health. They're also a good source of fiber which helps bowel movements and remove waste from the body. They're a good source of polyphenols, compounds that stimulate liver enzymes and detoxification.

- **Grapefruit** is rich in vitamin C, which helps protect the liver from oxidative stress; naringenin, a flavonoid that helps the liver to burn fat and prevents fatty liver; limonoids, compounds that stimulate the liver to produce enzymes that aid detoxification; pectin, a type of fiber that removes toxins from the gastrointestinal tract, and glutathione, the most potent antioxidant involved in liver health and detoxification.

- **Lemons** like grapefruit, lemons are high in vitamin C, can stimulate the liver to produce bile which helps flush toxins from the body, are high in limonene which supports phase 2 of biotransformation, and contain pectin, a soluble fiber that supports gut health.

- **Beets** are high in betalains, a crimson-colored antioxidant that reduces inflammation and oxidative stress in the liver. They're also high in betaine, a compound involved in the methylation process which converts chemicals into non-toxic, water-soluble substances for excretion. Beets are high in folate (B9), a B vitamin that supports the methylation process and liver detoxification. They're also high in fiber, which can help digestion and regulate bowel movements making it easier to eliminate toxins from the body.

- **Carrots** contain beta-carotene, an antioxidant that protects the liver from oxidative stress. They're also high in vitamin C, flavonoids, fiber, and potassium, all important for a healthy liver.

- **Bitter Greens** such as mustard, radicchio, dandelion, arugula, endive, kale, and sweet charge are high in several nutrients that support detoxification. They help stimulate bile, a substance the liver produces that helps remove waste from the body. They're rich in antioxidants like vitamins C and E and beta-carotene, which help neutralize free radicals. Bitter greens are high in fiber, promote regular bowel movements, and contain health-promoting phytonutrients. Bitter greens also promote glutathione production, the master antioxidant involved in detoxification.

- **Leafy Greens** are high in chlorophyll, a pigment that binds with environmental toxins and helps remove them from the body. They're also high in fiber, encouraging eliminating and removing waste and toxins from the body. Leafy greens are high in antioxidants that neutralize free radicals and folate, and magnesium which support liver detoxification. The cruciferous leafy greens are high in glucosinolates which break down into other compounds that stimulate the detoxifying liver enzymes. Leafy greens are associated with a lower risk of certain cancers.

- **Apples** contain pectin, a type of fiber that binds to toxins in the digestive tract and facilitates removal. They also contain phytochemicals such as quercetin, catechins, phloridzin, and chlorogenic acid that fight oxidative stress and protect the liver. Apples are a good source of malic acid, which thins and increases the movement of bile. They're also a good source of vitamin C, which protects the liver from damage and is involved in the production of glutathione, the most potent antioxidant in the body.

- **Avocados** are rich in healthy monounsaturated fats, which can reduce harmful cholesterol levels and decrease the risk of liver disease. Avocados contain antioxidants such as glutathione and vitamins C and E, protecting the liver from damage. They're high in fiber which helps to keep digestion healthy and the bowels moving.

- **Olive Oil** is rich in monounsaturated fatty acids, such as oleic acid, that help lower bad cholesterol and reduce the risk of fatty liver disease. It contains polyphenols, powerful antioxidants that protect against cellular damage and reduce inflammation and oxidative stress. Olive oil stimulates the production of liver enzymes that break down toxins and bile, crucial for removing waste from the liver.

- **Ginger** is rich in antioxidants that neutralize free radicals and reduce oxidative stress. It contains gingerols and shogaols, compounds that lower inflammation and support the liver's health. It improves the flow of bile and lipid metabolism, reducing the risk of non-alcoholic fatty liver diseases, and may boost the production of enzymes used in the detoxification process.

EAT LOTS OF FIBER

Fiber is a critical nutrient for detoxification and elimination. It binds to toxins, prevents them from being reabsorbed into the bloodstream, and removes them from the body. Fiber also promotes regular bowel movements and keeps the digestive system healthy. Fiber is a prebiotic, meaning it feeds the good bacteria in the gut that help break down toxins and remove them from the body.[29]

Good sources of fiber include fruit, whole grains, vegetables, legumes, nuts, and seeds. If you're not used to eating fiber, you may experience gas and bloating when you first start eating it. Start slow and gradually increase the amount daily. Fiber can be constipating if you're not consuming enough liquids. Be sure to drink more water as you increase your fiber intake to prevent constipation.

EAT ORGANIC WHENEVER POSSIBLE

Conventional foods have been heavily sprayed with pesticides in order to increase crop production. However, this comes with a price. The liver has to break down all the chemicals in order to extract them from the body. Eating foods sprayed with pesticides once in a while may not be a big deal, but consistent exposure can place a burden on the liver leading to inflammation, oxidative stress, and the accumulation of harmful substances in the body.[30]

Some studies have shown plants sprayed with pesticides don't make as many of the health promoting phytonutrients that support detoxification pathways.[31] Eating organic is important because it not only minimizes the extra toxic burden coming in, but you'll also get more phytonutrients that aid in the detoxification process. This is like a double benefit. If conventional is your only option, wash and scrub your produce to remove as much pesticides as possible.

GIVE YOUR GUT A BREAK

While the thought of fasting might initially seem daunting, the potential benefits to your body's detoxification process can be significant. Fasting doesn't mean going days without food; instead, it's about creating a consistent cycle between eating and not eating—referred to as your 'eating window' and 'fasting window.'

For beginners, I recommend starting with a balanced 12-hour cycle. This means if you finish dinner at 8 pm, you'll have your next meal at 8 am. What's great about this approach is its flexibility. Over time, you can adjust these windows based on your comfort and health goals. Some benefits you might experience include:

- Improved digestion
- Reduced bloating
- Enhanced energy levels
- Decreased pain and inflammation
- A better-fitting wardrobe

The magic behind fasting lies in its ability to give our digestive system a break, allowing our body to eliminate waste efficiently. It can also regulate blood sugar levels, boost metabolic health, and stimulate our liver to process toxins.

Begin by gradually shortening your eating window by 30 minutes daily until you reach the 12-hour mark. From there, adjust as you see fit, whether it's a 12:12, 14:10, or 16:8 ratio. Remember, everyone's body is different—find a rhythm that suits yours. If you have any health concerns, always consult a medical professional before fasting.

BOOST WITH SUPPLEMENTS

Adding supplements can be a great way to support the body's natural detoxification process. You can get many of these nutrients from an organic whole foods diet. However, there are many reasons to supplement.

Unfortunately, due to modern farming practices, many soils are depleted of essential nutrients leading to less nutrient-dense crops.[32] Some people have problems with their digestion and can't absorb nutrients from food.[33] Others have dysbiosis, a fancy term for an imbalance of good and bad gut bacteria contributing to nutrient deficiencies.[34] Stress, overwork, lack of sleep, poor diet, or exposure to more toxins can increase the body's need for nutrients.

The following is a list of supplements that support detoxification. However, always consult your healthcare provider before adding any new supplements to your diet.

- **Vitamin C** is not only a vitamin; it's a potent antioxidant that helps neutralize harmful chemicals in the body and reduce oxidative stress. It boosts glutathione levels and is involved in collagen production, which maintains the health and integrity of liver tissue. Vitamin C supports the immune system, indirectly supporting the liver, and prevents fat accumulation in the liver.

- **Vitamin E** is a powerful antioxidant that neutralizes chemicals and reduces oxidative stress. It protects against liver disease, boosts the immune system, and supports the health of the cell membrane protecting liver cells from oxidative damage.

- **Selenium** is a trace mineral that supports liver enzyme function and protects against liver disease by reducing inflammation, boosting antioxidant activity, and regulating the immune system.

- **Zinc** is a trace mineral that acts as an antioxidant and anti-inflammatory; it reduces inflammation and oxidative stress, supports liver enzyme function, protects against liver disease, and supports cell membrane stability.

- **Choline** aids in the transportation of fats out of the liver, preventing fatty liver disease. It helps to convert the harmful amino acid homocysteine into a benign substance. It helps maintain the cell's membrane, aids in the process of methylation, and is involved in the production of glutathione, the most potent antioxidant in the body.

- **Glutathione** is the master antioxidant because it's so good at neutralizing and eliminating toxins from the body. Foods rich in sulfur, such as garlic, onions, cruciferous vegetables, and eggs, contain glutathione.
- **N-acetyl cysteine (NAC)** is an amino acid involved in glutathione production. It provides protection against damage from toxins and drugs, aids in the management of liver disease, reduces inflammation, and promotes overall liver health.
- **Alpha-Lipoic Acid (ALA)** is a powerful antioxidant that protects the liver from damage by reducing inflammation and improving insulin sensitivity. It also acts as a mild metal chelator, binding to metals that could produce harmful free radicals
- **Antioxidants** like vitamins C and E and the minerals selenium and zinc aid in detoxification and protect cells from oxidative stress. Find them in citrus fruits, berries, nuts, and seeds contain antioxidants.
- **Magnesium** is high in nuts, seeds, leafy greens, and whole grains. It's a mineral that supports detoxification and other chemical processes in the body.
- **Omega-3 fatty acids** from fatty fish, flax, and chia seeds reduce inflammation and support cellular health, making detoxification a better experience.
- **Resveratrol** is a potent antioxidant that can neutralize harmful free radicals in the liver and reduce oxidative

stress. It's anti-inflammatory and protects the liver from damage and dysfunction.

- **Curcumin** in turmeric is similar to resveratrol because it's a powerful antioxidant that neutralizes harmful free radicals and reduces oxidative stress. It's also anti-inflammatory and boosts glutathione activity, protecting against fatty liver disease by reducing fat accumulation and inflammation in the liver. It may have anticancer properties and slow the progress of liver cancer.

- **B vitamins**, especially B6, B9 (folate), and B12, are involved in liver biotransformation and assist in the methylation process. Up your intake of leafy greens, whole grains, legumes, and animal products.

- **Chlorella** is a type of algae that binds to heavy metals like lead, mercury, cadmium, and other toxins and pulls them out of the body. It's also rich in antioxidants such as chlorophyll, vitamin C, beta-carotene, lycopene, and lutein which support the liver by neutralizing free radicals and reducing oxidative stress. Chlorella is fiber-rich, so it can help digestion and regulate bowel movements. Some studies suggest it's suitable for the immune system and can support its ability to fight infections and eliminate waste products.

- **Probiotics** may help to protect against liver disease through the gut-liver axis; they can reduce overall inflammation and decrease pro-inflammatory cytokines.

- **Amino acids** such as glutamine, glycine, taurine, glutamic acid, methionine, cysteine, and arginine are the building blocks of molecules and proteins involved in the detoxification process. They support the production of glutathione and aid in the methylation process. They help transform toxic substances into non-toxic metabolites that the body can safely excrete.

- **Milk Thistle** is a flowering herb that contains a group of antioxidants called silymarin. Silymarin blocks toxins from entering liver cells and stimulates their regeneration. Milk thistle fights oxidative stress, lowers inflammation, and boosts glutathione levels.

- **Dandelion root** contains an array of antioxidants that neutralize free radicals reduce harmful free radicals, and reduce oxidative stress. It enhances bile flow, supports fat digestion, and helps eliminate waste from the body. It's a diuretic that helps eliminate toxins through increased urine output.

- **Nettle** has a diuretic effect which aids in flushing waste products out of the body. It supports kidney and liver function, lowers inflammation, and contains antioxidants that protect the body from free radicals and oxidative stress.

- **Fiber** supports liver detoxification by adding bulk to the stool, promoting the removal of waste and toxins from the body. It binds to toxins in the digestive tract and can prevent them from being reabsorbed into the bloodstream. Fiber feeds the good gut bacteria essential for optimal liver function and detoxification. Fiber also reduces fat accumulation in the liver and helps to regulate cholesterol levels, so there's less burden on the liver.

CUT OUT LIVER-HARMING SUBSTANCES

When supporting the body's natural detoxification process, avoiding food and other substances that burden the liver is super important. Otherwise, all that effort you're putting in to clean out the body is only removing the surface or what you're currently putting in, not the deeper stuff. You're not improving your health if you continue to pile in toxins. Here's a list of foods to avoid while supporting your natural detoxification process;

- **Ultra-processed foods** are hight in chemicals that the liver has to break down. They're also full of unhealthy fats, sugars, and sodium. They're poor in nutrients such as fiber, antioxidants, vitamins, and minerals that your body needs to support detoxification. They decrease the amount of good bacteria needed to neutralize harmful toxins. They promote inflammation and oxidative stress, leading to an imbalance in hormones that play a role in detoxification.

- **Refined sugars** cause inflammation and metabolic syndrome, slowing the detoxification process. The liver has to process and break down fructose, and high levels can lead to overload and non-alcoholic fatty liver disease. Refined sugars throw off the balance of good and bad bacteria in the gut and deplete nutrients involved in detoxification, such as B vitamins, magnesium, and zinc. Avoid soda, fruit juice, or anything with high fructose corn syrup (HFCS).

- **Alcohol** is a toxin, and excessive use leads to liver damage. The liver has to work hard to detox alcohol. It depletes nutrients essential in detoxification, such as B vitamins and glutathione. Alcohol disrupts the balance of good and bad bacteria in the gut, can damage the gut lining, and increase permeability, allowing toxins to enter the bloodstream. Alcohol is also dehydrating, making it harder for the kidneys to filter out waste products from the blood.

- **Excess caffeine** leads to dehydration which slows down detoxification. Drink one full glass of water for every cup of coffee or other caffeine source you consume.

- **Unhealthy fats** such as refined vegetable oils (sunflower, corn, canola, soybean, cottonseed, grapeseed, and safflower) are high in omega-6 fatty acids. When consumed in large quantities promote inflammation and oxidative stress. Refined oils lack nutrients and contain chemicals from the refining process. Avoid trans fats and fried foods because they lead to inflammation and oxidative stress, damaging the liver and slowing down detoxification.

- **Processed meats** increase the body's overall toxic load. They contain harmful compounds like nitrates and nitrites that convert into nitrosamines, a potential carcinogen. They also promote inflammation and oxidative stress and decrease the beneficial bacteria in your gut.

- **Dairy products** can be hard to digest for some people. Lactose intolerance and casein sensitivity can cause digestive problems, inflammation, and impaired detoxification. Conventional dairy contains hormones and antibiotics that increase the toxic burden on the liver. Full-fat dairy products are high in saturated fats, raising cholesterol and impacting liver function when consumed excessively. Avoid dairy if you suspect you have an issue with it.

- **Conventional produce** is sprayed with pesticides which add to your body's toxic load. Pesticides have to be broken down by the liver. They stimulate the production of free radicals, unstable molecules that damage cells and contribute to oxidative stress. Pesticides disrupt the gut microbiome and lower the balance of good bacteria that assist in the breakdown and neutralization of chemicals. Eat organic whenever possible, especially foods from the dirty dozen list.

- **Artificial sweeteners and additives** interfere with your body's natural detoxification process and harm the gut. Artificial sweeteners and additives lead to dysbiosis, an imbalance in your gut microbiota. A healthy microbiome is crucial for healthy detoxification. They also affect insulin response and glucose metabolism and cause inflammation and oxidative stress.

DETOX

- **Smoking and recreational drug use** burden the liver by introducing harmful toxins that the liver has to break down. Smoking impairs the body's ability to detoxify itself, eventually leading to chronic diseases like emphysema, bronchitis, and lung cancer. Recreational drugs can damage the liver, kidneys, lungs, and other organs involved in detoxification. All drugs create inflammation and oxidative stress, which further hinders detoxification leading to chronic diseases.

- **Over-the-Counter Medications** such as acetaminophen (Tylenol), and non-steroidal anti-inflammatory drugs (NSAIDS), like ibuprofen and naproxen can lead to liver damage and block liver enzymes that metabolize other substances. This can lead to build up of toxic substances making it harder for the liver to do its job.

EXERCISE TO SUPPORT DETOXIFICATION

Exercise is more than just a way to look and feel better, it's also a major player in the body's natural detoxification process. Here's how;

- **Improves circulation** bringing oxygen and nutrients to every cell while simultaneously carrying away metabolic waste. Improved blood flow indirectly aids the liver and bolsters the kidneys by helping regulate blood pressure, manage cholesterol, and stabilize blood sugar levels.

- **Promotes sweating** which pushes waste products out through your skin. When we exercise, the body naturally heats up, causing the body to sweat.

- **Improves respiration** When we exercise, we tend to breathe faster and deeper, filling our lungs with fresh air while expelling carbon dioxide, a waste product of metabolism.

- **Improves digestion and promotes bowel movements** thus reducing the risk of constipation and the reabsorption of waste products.

The beauty of exercise is its versatility. Whether you're into cardiovascular routines, strength training, flexibility exercises, or focused breathing practices, each contributes to detoxification. The key is consistency. Even if it's just a brisk 20-minute walk, choose an activity you love and make it a regular part of your routine. The benefits for your body's detox system, and overall health, are undeniable.

PRIORITIZE SLEEP

Good sleep allows the body to repair, regenerate, and rebalance itself. We learned in the Sleep section that the brain's detoxification system works when we sleep. The liver is also affected by sleep and operates on a 24-hour cycle.

At night, when you're sleeping, the liver is busy neutralizing toxins, synthesizing proteins, and producing chemicals essential for digestion and other functions. There's also a reduction in inflammatory and stress hormones that interfere with the liver's ability to do its job. Inadequate sleep disrupts all these processes.

The brain and central nervous system (CNS) have their own cleaning mechanism called the glymphatic system. The glymphatic system primarily functions while we're sleeping. Like the lymphatic system, which uses vessels and lymph nodes to remove waste from the body, the glymphatic system removes harmful waste from the brain. Waste from brain cells builds up and can cause inflammation and lead to unwanted changes in the brain.

Consistently not sleeping may increase your risk of developing a neurodegenerative disease like Alzheimer's and Parkinson's.[35] Prioritizing adequate and good-quality sleep is crucial to your well-being. Refer to the SLEEP section for ways to get better sleep.

FIND WAYS TO UNWIND

Stress, whether it's psychological, physical, or chronic, can have detrimental effects on the liver and its detoxification functions. It causes your body to release stress hormones that promote inflammation, oxidative stress, and weight gain.

Stress also lowers your immune system, meaning your body has more difficulty fighting infections, including those targeting the liver. Chronic stress can lead to poor sleep, bad diet, and reduced physical activity, hindering the liver's ability to detox.

While the body is designed to handle short-term stress effectively, it's not equipped to be constantly stressed. Stress can be managed through relaxation techniques, exercise, adequate sleep, eating a balanced diet, connecting with loved ones, and engaging in activities that bring you joy.

DRY BRUSH YOUR SKIN

Dry brushing may sound strange, but it can be one of the most invigorating ways to start your day. The soft, natural bristles stimulate the skin, promoting circulation of the cardiovascular and lymphatic systems.

The lymphatic system is a network of vessels directly below the skin that remove toxins and waste products from the body. Unlike the cardiovascular system, which uses the heart to pump blood throughout the body continuously, the lymphatic system has no pump and relies on physical movement. Hence, it's prone to stagnation.

Sluggish lymph wasn't a problem for our ancestors, who spent most of the day moving, but modern people spend a lot of time sitting in the same position, leading to the buildup of fluid and waste products.

Dry brushing moves the fluid and promotes the drainage of waste. It also exfoliates the skin and opens the pores, which leaves you soft and silky. Dry brushing is excellent before the sauna because it preps the skin for better perspiration, aiding in detoxification. How do you dry brush?

- **Get a brush:** Nowadays, there are plenty of dry brushes on Amazon. Be sure to pick one with natural, soft-fiber bristles and a long handle to reach your back.

- **Start at your feet**: Begin at your feet and gently brush upwards towards your knees. In general, you always want to be brushing in the direction of your heart. Be sure to get all areas of your lower legs, paying particular attention to the back of your knees.

- **Work Your Way Up:** Continue brushing your entire leg using upward strokes until you reach your inguinal area. Brush your buttocks, pelvic area, and back, always brushing toward the heart.

- **Move to your Hands:** Brush your arms entirely, starting with your hands and working towards your heart.

- **Avoid Sensitive Areas:** Avoid brushing over broken skin, nipples, and sensitive, red, infected areas, as this could cause irritation.

- **Avoid the Face:** Don't brush your face unless you have a brush made for the face. A regular dry brush is too rough for the delicate skin on the face.

- **Shower & Moisturize:** After dry brushing, jump in the shower to rinse off the dead skin cells. Finish up with a moisturizer to nourish and hydrate the skin.

- **Clean the Brush:** Use mild soap and warm water to remove the dead skin cells from your brush.

Dry brushing may not have a lot of research behind it, but there is a lot of anecdotal evidence, meaning people have found that it works for them despite not being backed by evidence. So go ahead and try it. If anything, you'll feel refreshed from the increased circulation and have smoother skin.

GET A MASSAGE

Massage is an ancient healing technique used for thousands of years to relieve pain and promote health. Like dry brushing, massage is a great way to stimulate the lymphatic and cardiovascular systems.

Abdominal massage, in particular, can get the digestive organs going and encourage bowel movements. Be sure to drink plenty of water before and after a massage to help with this process and alleviate dehydration.

You can get a massage or perform self-massage using the same steps as dry brushing. Warm some massage oil between your hands and begin massaging from your feet, gradually working your way up your body.

SIT IN A SAUNA

Sitting in a sauna is one of the best ways to enhance the body's natural detoxification process. The warmth elevates your body's temperature, triggering a bout of perspiration and allowing toxins to leave the body through the skin. The sauna's heat improves circulation, helping deliver nutrients and remove unwanted waste products from the body.

While Finland holds the prize for modern sauna use, heat therapy has a rich history and has been integral to various cultures for thousands of years. Native Americans used sweat lodges for purification and spiritual ceremonies. Romans were famous for bathhouses and the laconicum, their version of a sauna. Russians have "banyas," a type of bathhouse with a steam room, washing room, and relaxation area. Korean bathhouses include hot tubs, saunas, and steam rooms. Japan has a tradition of bathing in hot springs and steam bathing.

Traditional saunas heat the air around you, which heats your body from the outside in and promotes sweating. They generally use dry heat and stick to temperatures around 150 to 195 F.

Infrared saunas use infrared light waves to heat your body from the inside out. The heat from infrared light waves penetrates deeper, which induces a more vigorous sweat at lower temperatures, generally 120 to 150 F. Infrared saunas are more comfortable, so you can stay in them for longer periods.

The heat from infrared saunas mimics a fever which kills microbes. To enhance the detoxifying benefits of a sauna, try dry brushing, massage, or exercising beforehand. Be sure to rinse off afterward to remove any toxins from the skin.

Sitting in the sauna can be a relaxing and stress-reducing activity. However, start slow with shorter sessions and listen to your body. Overuse can lead to dehydration and other heat-related conditions. If you're pregnant or have a health condition, consult your healthcare provider before using the sauna.

TAKE AN EPSOM SALT BATH

Taking an Epsom salt bath is one of my favorite ways to detox. The warm water is relaxing and helps to open up the pores, which helps to absorb the salts through the skin. Warm baths also support the lymphatic system, which helps move toxins out of the body.

Epsom salt is made out of magnesium sulfate. When absorbed by the skin, magnesium can support various bodily functions, including muscle relaxation and removing toxins. Magnesium promotes restful sleep, which, as we learned above, is needed for overall detoxification.

Epsom salt contains sulfur, which is needed for phase 2 liver biotransformation and removing harmful substances from the body. It's also essential for synthesizing glutathione, one of the body's most potent antioxidants and detoxifiers.

To take an Epsom salt bath:

- Fill the tub with warm water and add 1 - 2 cups of Epsom salt. You might need to add more Epsom salt if you have a large tub.
- Make sure the salts are thoroughly dissolved to maximize the detoxification potential.

DETOX

- Try adding a few drops of your favorite relaxing essential oils for an added treat. Lavender is known to be relaxing.

- Soak for 20 minutes, then rinse off to remove any salts from your skin.

- Be sure to drink plenty of water before and after the bath to support detoxification and to ensure you don't get dehydrated.

USE AN AIR PURIFIER

An air purifier might be the missing link to your mysterious allergies and breathing problems. They help reduce the number of pollutants and contaminants in your home by using filters that capture and trap particles flying around in the air that would otherwise end up in your lungs. Air purifiers limit exposure to allergies like pollen, mold spores, dust, and pet dander.

If your purifier contains a carbon filter, it can also help reduce your exposure to volatile organic compounds (VOCs), which are gasses emitted from many household products, including paints, cleaning supplies, and cosmetics. Carbon filters also remove odors and smoke from the air.

Air purifiers with ultraviolet (UV) lights can kill or deactivate airborne pathogens like bacteria, viruses, and mold. This can lower your microbial load, reducing your risk of getting sick.

Be sure to get an air purifier large enough to filter your home, or invest in smaller ones for each room. The only downside is remembering to change the filters regularly. One way to remedy this is to put it on your calendar so when the time comes, you're prepared.

INVEST IN A WATER FILTER

While tap water may be safe to drink according to your city's water supplier, it still contains pharmaceuticals and other chemicals. Here's how a good filtration system can limit your exposure to harmful substances;

- **Removes Heavy Metals:** A good filtration system can remove heavy metals like lead, mercury, arsenic, and cadmium. Chronic exposure to these metals can harm the nervous system.

- **Eliminates Chlorine and Chloramine:** Chlorine and chloramine are chemicals frequently added to municipal water supplies to kill pathogens. The downside is that they can also alter your gut microbiome by killing good bacteria.

- **Reduces Organic Chemicals:** A filtration system can reduce or eliminate VOCs and other synthetic chemicals.

- **Reduces Endocrine Disruptors:** Endocrine disruptors such as bisphenol A (BPA) and phthalates have been found in tap water. These chemicals interfere with the body's hormonal system and are linked to reproductive disorders.

- **Blocks Pathogens:** A filtration system can trap bacteria, viruses, parasites, and other pathogens that could harm your body.

- **Supports Cellular Health:** Filtration systems support cellular health by lessening the burden that toxins place on the body.

- **Reduces Skin Exposure:** Your skin absorbs substances through shower and bath water. A whole house filtration system can protect your skin and reduce exposure.

Not all water filtration systems work the same. The type of filter and its specifications determine which contaminants are removed. You must determine which contaminants are in your water and select a filtration system that addresses those concerns. You can find this information on your city's water supplier website or call and ask them for this information. You can also test your water using test strips that can be found on amazon.

Now that you know a little more about how your body naturally gets rid of harmful substances, you can nudge it along by consuming the right food and nutrients, exercising, staying hydrated, getting adequate sleep, finding ways to unwind, and avoiding anything that makes the liver sluggish.

Just like anything else in this book, start slow. Pick one or two things you think will be the easiest to change. Over time, you can go down the list and continue improving your well-being in phases.

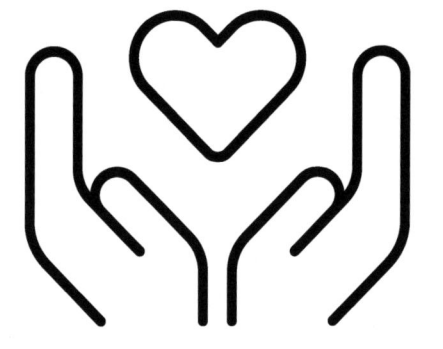

Connect

Community is the foundation upon which we build our lives.
~ Bryant McGill

I'm sure you've heard of the infamous phrase, "You are what you eat." It's a cute way of saying your food affects your overall health. But have you heard the phrase, "You are who you hang out with?" It implies that your social circle influences your behavior, attitudes, choices, and identity.

On a superficial level, this makes sense. We tend to be drawn to people who think like ourselves, have the same point of view, and enjoy the same type of entertainment.

However, did you know the people you're closest to influence your health and even how long you live?[1]

A study out of Harvard found that if your friends, family, or spouse become overweight, you are likely to become overweight as well.[2] This is called network phenomena and suggests obesity is spread through social ties and behavior.

We tend to adopt the behaviors of our social networks, including eating habits, physical activity levels, and attitudes toward health.

If all your friends drink beer and eat burgers and french fries at the local pub every weekend, you'll likely do the same. If your friends are into hiking, smoothies, and self-improvement, you'll soon engage in those behaviors.

This is why it's so important to choose your community wisely. Your social fabric determines your success in life. If you have friends who encourage you to grow and be a better person, then it will be a lot easier to do so. Good social connections boost your mood, lower your blood pressure, and even extend your life.

A BRIEF HISTORY OF COMMUNITIES

In the book Sapiens: A Brief History of Humankind, Yuval Noah Harari argues that Sapiens are the only species that cooperate in large numbers.[3] It's what allowed us to come out of the caves and form tribes of like-minded people who learned to farm together, create tools and weapons, build homes, then towns, then large societies, and essentially dominate the world. We're also the only species able to use our imagination to create fictitious stories and bond over those stories. We have shared beliefs in imaginary things like money and government.

Communities are formed from various factors, including cultural identity, traditions, stories, shared beliefs, religion, interests, or geographical locations. They give their members a sense of belonging, safety, and support.

Nowadays, you can join just about any community with a click of your mouse. Technology has expanded our reach and ability to connect with like-minded individuals across the globe, transcending the geographical barriers that once kept us apart. Information sharing has become incredibly easy, with instant messaging, FaceTime, Zoom, and live streaming all at the tip of your fingers.

But even so, finding the right community can be challenging. You want to ensure your community supports and aligns with your values. Sometimes, it takes some experimentation, but once you know yourself and what you value, you can be more selective in who you allow in your life.

Here's how to build a strong community with an emphasis on living a longer and healthier life;

START WITH YOURSELF

*Yesterday I was clever, so I wanted to change the world.
Today I am wise, so I am changing myself.*
~ Rumi

The relationship you have with yourself is the single most important relationship you will have in your life. It is the foundation of all relationships that follow. You can not have a healthy relationship with another person until you have worked on the one with yourself. You have to understand your needs, desires, strengths, and weaknesses before you can expect anyone else to know these things about you.

I grew up in a dynamic family in Los Angeles, California. Being the fourth out of five children and the second daughter, there was nothing special about me and my place in the family. My parents were very active in the community. They were attentive parents but often overwhelmed by responsibilities. My older siblings all had strong personalities and dominated the house with a mixture of laughter and shouting matches. Although my birth order didn't give me special privileges, I always felt loved and cared for.

However, middle child syndrome was something I identified with for a long time. I didn't think I mattered much and, therefore, didn't put much effort into school exploring my interests or talents. My self-esteem wasn't the greatest, and I developed the bad habit of putting other people's needs before mine because I thought I wasn't important.

But that bad habit followed me through many relationships, and soon, I was resenting the people I loved for not reading my mind. Didn't they know my needs weren't being met?

When I finally caught on that the pattern of broken relationship after broken relationship had something to do with me, I swallowed my pride and began to work on myself. It wasn't easy, but mandatory if I was to become a better person.

Working on myself turned out to be the best decision I ever made. By giving myself the love and attention I deserved, I was able to grow out of those limiting childhood beliefs and develop healthy, loving relationships with not only myself, but my loved ones as well. It was incredibly freeing.

That one change birthed many others. When I started valuing and respecting myself, I realized the importance of self-care. I began eating healthier, saying no more, setting boundaries, and doing things I love, like cooking and going on long hikes in the mountains. Nurturing myself allowed me to heal and created a solid foundation to build future relationships.

Take a moment to answer the following questions about yourself;

- What are my needs?

- Do I actively seek out ways to satisfy my needs?

- What are my strengths and weaknesses?

- Do I let people know how I want to be treated?

- Is there anything that's holding me back?

- Am I living the life that I want to live, and if not, what changes could I make to redirect my life?

To build a stronger relationship with yourself, you need to practice self-awareness and compassion for yourself, set boundaries, teach people how to treat you, and prioritize your needs. Doing so sets the stage for all relationships that follow.

BEING WELL

NURTURE YOUR RELATIONSHIPS

*The grass isn't greener on the other side,
the grass is greener where it's watered.*

~ Fr. Dr. Charles Ara

My father, a marriage and family counselor, always emphasizes the importance of working on relationships. He believes that, like grass, if you want a relationship to last, you have to water it. One of the best ways to nurture your relationship is by practicing what he calls the 5As of healthy relationships: affection, appreciation, attention, acceptance, and availability. According to him, these elements are what keep relationships alive and thriving.

Affection is the emotional adhesive that creates a sense of closeness, showing your loved one you care beyond words. Whether it's a simple hug, a warm smile, a loving glance, or a caring check-in, affection strengthens the bond between two people. Reflect on how you show affection:

- In what ways do you express affection?
- What gestures make you feel most loved?
- Can you think of new ways to show your love?

Appreciation is the recognition of what your partner brings to the relationship. It makes your loved one feel seen and valued. Whether it's saying thank you for a meal they made or acknowledging their help, appreciation lessens the chance of taking each other for granted. Consider these points:

- What qualities in your loved ones are you truly grateful for?

- What do they do for you, big or small, that you can show appreciation for?

- Share them with your loved one and encourage them to do the same for you.

Attention is the genuine curiosity and commitment to being present in each other's lives. It involves active listening and engaging in conversations, which shows you value their thoughts and feelings. Think about your current listening habits:

- Are you actively listening when they are talking, or are you thinking about something else?

- Do you scroll on your phone in their presence, or do you give them the gift of your undivided attention?

- Next time they talk, don't interrupt; provide them with eye contact and your full attention.

- Reflect on how attention can deepen your understanding and connection with your loved one.

Acceptance is letting your loved one be who they are without judgment. Embracing each other's imperfections creates a safe space for authenticity without the fear of rejection. No one is perfect, and we all have flaws and traits that make us unique. Think about the following questions;

- In what ways do you show acceptance?

- Has there been a time you didn't feel accepted by your loved one?

- Has there been a time you didn't fully accept your loved one?

- How can you create a safe space to be fully authentic and accepted by each other?

Availability is making time for each other, whether it's a quick text or chat on the phone, an outing, or doing something they want to do. It's spending quality time together, not just sitting next to each other on the couch scrolling on your smartphones. It's being there for them when they need you. Ask yourself these questions:

- Do you answer your loved one's phone calls and texts?

- How often do they make time for you?

- Are you making quality time for your loved ones?

If you want loving relationships, then you need to actively work on them. The 5As provide a solid foundation to do just that, built on love, respect, and mutual understanding for one another.

NOTICE WHAT YOU LIKE

People are dynamic creatures full of traits, opinions, thoughts, and unique ways of doing things. If you want a healthy relationship, focus more on what you like about the other person rather than what you don't. If you're constantly nitpicking their faults, you won't be able to see their positive traits. I'm not saying you should stick around in an abusive relationship, but even good, well-meaning people might annoy you from time to time.

Someone you love may be messy, talk too loud, or have an annoying laugh, but they can be fun, share your views on life, and be there for you when needed. Here are some ways to get yourself out of a cycle of fault-finding;

- Remind yourself of their strengths. What unique qualities do they have that you admire and appreciate?

- Put yourself in their shoes. Why might they have these traits? Understanding their perspective can help you appreciate their way of doing things.

- Don't talk about your differences. If you have different political views, avoid talking about politics. Stick to lighter conversations or areas that you agree on.

- Give them compliments. Telling them what you like makes them feel good, trains your brain to see what you like, and reinforces your positive view of them.

Focusing on what you like leads to fewer arguments and encourages a deeper and more meaningful relationship. You not only reduce conflicts but build stronger bonds that last a lifetime.

MAKE NEW CONNECTIONS

Friendship is born at that moment when one person says to another, 'What! You too? I thought I was the only one.

~ C.S. Lewis

While it's important to work on and enjoy the company you already have, it's equally important to continue making new friends. Why? Because life is long, and you'll likely change multiple times throughout the course of it.

Your interests will change, your habits change, and so forth. Evolution is a normal part of life, and new people satisfy different parts of you. You become each other's teachers, introducing fresh perspectives you'd otherwise not take the time to learn about.

Venturing out to make new friends can be an exciting and daunting adventure. You can make new friends through mutual friends and family members, clubs, church, workshops, school, work, workout studios, and social platforms that contain communities of like-minded individuals. When looking for new friends, ask yourself the following questions;

- What qualities do I value in a friend?
- What are my boundaries?
- Am I looking for close friendships or a broader social circle?
- Where can I go to meet new people?

CONNECT

- What online groups can I join to meet new people?

While the avenues to meet new people are numerous, sometimes friendships form spontaneously. Knowing yourself and what you value can significantly enhance your ability to connect and lead to unexpected, rewarding, and lifelong friendships.

PICK YOUR BATTLES

No matter how well two people get along, there are going to be disagreements. It's unrealistic to think you'll agree on everything with everyone. However, this doesn't mean your differing views have to turn into a full-fledged argument. It's healthy to have people with different views in your life, even if you think they are entirely wrong. Instead of arguing, I encourage you to pick your battles. What is really worth having a shouting match over? Often it's better to let things go and move on. Constantly arguing over trivial matters doesn't improve the quality of anyone's life or relationship. Before you get into an argument, pause and consider these questions:

- Does it really matter?
- Will it matter tomorrow or a year from now?
- Do I need to be right? If so, why?
- Will arguing make a difference?
- Is it worth the heartache it will cause the other person?

BEING WELL

- Can I sleep on it first before bringing it up?

- How would I want someone to bring up a difficult conversation with me?

If you do decide to discuss the matter, consider approaching it in a non-confrontational way. People often become defensive when confronted, triggering that fight-or-flight response. It's hard to think rationally when your body thinks a tiger is chasing it.

To get more out of the conversation, do it when you're both calm and in a distraction free environment. Express your feelings without blaming the other person, use clear and concise words, actively listen to their point of view, and learn to be empathic. If you can focus on finding a solution rather than blame, you are far more likely to have a positive outcome.

RETHINK YOUR TOP 5

You are the average of the five people you spend the most time with.

~ Jim Rohn

The quote above is based on the law of averages, a statistical principle suggesting random events even out within a small sample. In other words, the patterns and habits of the top five people you hang out with rub off on you, so it's important to choose them wisely. If you spend a lot of time with happy, successful, and motivated people, you are more likely to become happy, successful, and motivated as well.

If you want to learn to speak French, spend time with people who speak French. If you want to learn to play guitar, spend time with people who play guitar. If you want to laugh more, spend time with people with a sense of humor. If you want to get over a chronic disease, seek out a support system of people who overcame that disease.

Write down the names of the top five people you associate with and ask yourself the following questions about each of them;

- Do they share my values and goals?
- Am I inspired by their achievements?
- Do they encourage me to be the best I can be?
- How do they make me feel when I'm in their presence?
- Is there anyone else I'd rather spend my time with who would be a positive influence?

Once you have these questions answered you can reevaluate your relationships and seek out new ones if needed.

BE THE INFLUENCER

Needing to let go of bad habits sometimes means letting go of a group of people those habits are associated with. This is where most people struggle because they don't want to give up their meaningful friendships, especially if the alternative is solitude.

However, you may not have to let go of them completely. You can be the shining star, introducing your group to healthier habits. You can be the person who brings healthy food or mocktails to the party or arranges a game of pickleball or cards instead of a night out at the bar.

Some friends might be curious and willing to join your health crusade. Maybe they've been itching for a change but didn't know how to make it happen. As you become healthier, lose weight, and seem happier or more energetic, they'll be inspired and want that for themselves.

As time passes and your new, healthier habits solidify, it may be easier to hang out with friends without returning to your self-defeating habits. Maybe you can go to the bar without ordering beer and a plate of fried food and instead order the Liquid Death, aka sparkling water, grilled chicken strips, and a salad.

But this requires self-awareness, discipline, and honesty. If you can't hang out with those people without going down a rabbit hole of bad habits, trust that the universe will take care of you. Find out where the healthy people in your area are and hang out there. They exist and are probably more than happy to have you join their team. Ask yourself these questions and answer them honestly;

- Do my friends support my decision to get healthier?
- Would they be open to doing healthy activities with me?

CONNECT

- Have they expressed a desire to become healthier as well?

- Can I hangout with them without engaging in unhealthy activities?

Ultimately, the path to better health sometimes means finding a new community that supports your growth. It requires courage, a deep desire for change, and trust that everything will turn out okay. Those who genuinely support your development and want the best for you will support you and may even join you on your journey.

PULL THE WEEDS

Like pulling weeds from the garden, removing negative people from your life allows your social garden to flourish and thrive. Be selective and seek out people who inspire you. This next exercise is inspired by Jack Canfield in his book, The Success Principles.

Make a list of all the people you spend time with regularly. Include friends, coworkers, family members, neighbors, acquaintances, and members of your religious or other organizations.

Next, put a plus (+) or minus (-) sign beside their names. Put a plus sign next to the people you feel good or neutral around. These people make you laugh, lift your spirits, encourage you to be your best, or are generally positive.

BEING WELL

Put a minus sign next to those you don't feel good around. Maybe they're always complaining or gossiping, putting you or others down, or undermining your success. Be honest with yourself; if someone is important to you but doesn't make you feel good, they still get the minus next to their name.

Next comes the hard part—stop spending time with the people who have a minus sign by their name. I realize if it's your spouse or coworker, you can't completely stop spending time with them. However, you should seriously consider taking breaks. The amount of free time we have during the day is limited—there's no reason to spend it with people who bring tension and conflict to your life.

Once you get the courage to do this, your life feels much lighter without all the negativity.

STAY IN TOUCH

We can live without religion and meditation, but we cannot survive without human affection.
~ The Dalai Lama

One of the most haunting legacies of the COVID-19 pandemic was the loneliness that resulted from the lockdowns and social isolation. As businesses closed and streets emptied, many were trapped in their homes alone without the warmth of human connection.

CONNECT

We saw a surge of ailments as people's mental and physical health broke down. The rates of depression, anxiety, and post-traumatic stress disorder (PTSD) increased, as well as obesity, heart disease, stroke, type 2 diabetes, addiction, suicide, dementia, and premature death.[4]

But the good news was that people learned to use Zoom and other platforms to stay connected. It didn't replace the need for in-person contact, but it did help take the edge off and offer a digital way to stay connected.

Social connections provide comfort, belonging, and emotional support during difficult times. Just having that one person to spill your heart out to can be the difference between drowning and staying afloat.

Staying connected can be as simple as texting or calling a friend, scheduling that lunch date, getting coffee or going for a walk with a loved one, or eating a home-cooked meal together. What ways do you stay connected?

Now that you know the foundations of healthy relationships, you can go out and start implementing them right away. Remember to start with yourself so you know who you are and your needs before entering into lifelong relationships. This simple step can save you years of heartache.

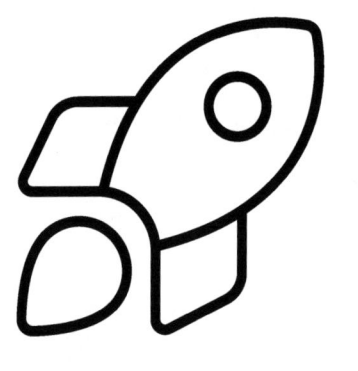

Pursue

Live each day based on your clearly defined values, purposes, and goals.

~ Dr. Daniel Amen

Have you ever thought about what your purpose is in life? Why are you here, and what can you do to make this world better? For some, the answer strikes like lightning. They know exactly their purpose and have been on a mission to complete their destiny since day one.

But for many, the answer to these questions is muffled. Maybe you haven't even considered your purpose. Or you thought you knew, but after dabbling around, you still haven't found something that fits. We all want to be happy and live a meaningful life, but many have no idea how to make this possible.

Don't stress. Wherever you are on this journey is exactly where you're supposed to be. Finding your purpose isn't a race with an end goal; it's a continual process of self-discovery where you use your internal compass as a guide. Some of us have one true purpose for being here. For others, it changes and morphs over time.

Ikigai (pronounced ee-kee-guy) is a Japanese concept that roughly translates to "a reason for being." I like to think of it like your purpose on steroids because it's more than doing what you're passionate about. It's the junction where doing what you love, what you are good at, what the world needs, and what you can be paid for meets.

WHY FIND YOUR IKIGAI?

The only way to do great work is to love what you do. If you haven't found it yet, keep looking. Don't settle.

~ Steve Jobs

When was the last time you felt joy and excitement about something you were about to do? Like you couldn't wait to get out of bed so you could do that thing you're passionate about?

If you're like most adults, you probably dread getting out of bed because it means you have to go to work and fulfill obligations. But wouldn't it be better to wake up and look forward to your work and responsibilities? Finding your Ikigai can bring back that lust for life you felt as a kid.

And Ikigai doesn't just bring you joy; it is a foundation of well-being because it encourages you to live a healthier life.

PURSUE

Those living in Okinawa, Japan, where the concept of Ikigai originated, credit their long, healthy lives to Ikigai. Okinawa is a Bluezone and home to many centenarians, where many work well into their 90s. Having a sense of purpose has been linked to reduced chronic disease, better cognitive function and emotional health, stronger social connections, and lower rates of stress.[1] A life led by purpose benefits the mind, body, and spirit.

Your Ikigai is very personal to you; however, the world needs you to find it just as much as you do. People who are passionate, living meaningful lives, and making a difference tend to glow and radiate positivity. They're like magnets. They make other people want to be better as well. In a sense, by finding your Ikigai and truly being happy, you're lifting the entire vibration of the planet. No pressure. :)

Finding your Ikigai comes down to four simple question;

1. What do you love to do?

2. What does the world need?

3. What are you good at?

4. What can you get paid to do?

WHAT DO YOU LOVE TO DO?

One of the first steps in finding your Ikigai is figuring out what you love doing. We all love doing something, so if something doesn't come to mind right away pause and ask yourself these questions;

- What makes me feel alive, content, or fulfilled?
- What topics do I love learning about?
- What do I never get bored of doing?
- What gets me excited?
- What keeps pulling me back in?
- What brings me to a flow state where I go so deep that I forget to eat and lose track of time?
- Go back to your childhood memories. What did you love to do then?
- What did your parents say you always loved doing?

Don't be afraid to ask friends and family members for ideas. They've probably spent enough time with you to provide insight into what you like doing.

It's okay not to know what you love to do. In this case, you have to be willing to try new things. Travel, take classes and workshops, and engage in activities that expose you to different experiences. Meditation quiets the background noise so you can hear your inner voice and discover what you truly love doing.

You may find that what you love is dynamic and changes over time. The point is to stay curious, regularly check in with yourself, and be willing to try new things.

PURSUE

Make a list of five or more things that you love doing. For example, I love cooking, writing, talking and reading about health, daydreaming, spending time out in nature, listening to health podcasts, and learning technology.

WHAT DOES THE WORLD NEED?

This one might be a little more tricky because it requires looking outside yourself. You're being asked to think about what others need, not just yourself. But keep in mind that happiness also comes from feeling valued by others. Helping the world can bring you as much joy as doing what you love.

To make it feel more personal, you can think about what the people in your immediate world need, the people in your state, town, or community that you live and work in. Ask yourself these questions;

- What are the people in my community like?
- What do they need?
- What will create a positive effect on my immediate community?
- What community or global issues concern me the most?
- Where do I notice gaps in services or products?
- What issues get me excited to think about?

- What problems am I interested in solving, and how can my skills, knowledge base, and talents solve these problems?

Finding what the world needs requires you to stay informed and up to date. It requires you to have conversations and network with people from diverse backgrounds and professions. Volunteering is another way to engage and get a feel for your community's needs. For example, if you want an online business, get to know the platform you wish to use, research trends in your niche, create surveys, and ask for feedback.

Make a list of five things you think the world needs and feel you're capable of addressing. For example, I think the world needs better healthcare, cooking shows that address healthier cooking methods and recipes, more creative outlets, a way to reconnect to nature, and more people teaching the benefits of self-care.

WHAT ARE YOU GOOD AT?

I like to include "what are you *willing* to get good at" in this one because people don't always know what they're good at. They're shadowed by limiting beliefs and societal expectations that they haven't had an opportunity to explore their talents. Ask yourself these questions;

- What do I know I'm good at?
- What do people ask me to help them with?

PURSUE

- What have I studied and consider myself educated in?
- What skills have I been practicing or mastered?
- What classes did I get good grades in at school?
- What comes naturally and easily to me?
- Is there anything I'm not great at now but are willing to put the time and effort into improving?
- What can I become good at with practice?

You don't have to be good at it now, but you do have to be willing to learn new things and overcome obstacles.

List five things you're good at and are willing to get good at. I am good at acupuncture, nutrition, functional medicine, giving health advice, cooking healthy food, and reading and writing about health. I could learn how to code and create a YouTube channel and a podcast to share my expertise with more people.

WHAT CAN YOU GET PAID FOR?

There are thousands of jobs and professions in this world. The good news is that many of them will align with your Ikigai. Figuring out what you can get paid for requires market research, self-assessment, and experimentation.

Given what you love, what you're good at, and what the world needs, what could you get paid for doing? Ask yourself these questions;

BEING WELL

- What services or products can I earn money with?
- Which of my skills and passions are in demand?
- What jobs align with my interests?
- How have others used similar skills to make money?
- How can I market my skills to potential employers?
- What will pay well enough to live comfortably in my town? Someone living in New York City will have to make more money than someone living in a rural town.

List five things you can get paid for based on your skills and expertise. Mine are acupuncture, functional medicine, writing, nutritional advice, etc.

TAKE ACTION

He who has a why to live can bear almost any how.
~ Friedrich Nietzsche

Hooray, you found your Ikigai! Now what? Now, you take action to turn it into reality. Living a purposeful life doesn't mean you don't have to work, but your work will be more exciting, enjoyable, and meaningful to you.

First and foremost, reflect on your Ikigai and really get clear on your vision. Visualize what you want to help turn it into realty. Think about what you can realistically achieve in the near and distant future, then write it all down. Brain dump everything that comes to mind and use this as your roadmap as you navigate through the process.

One of the best ways to achieve your goals is using the SMART format. SMART stands for specific, measurable, achievable, relevant, and time-bound. It helps you organize your goals and set realistic expectations of how and when to achieve them. Here's an example of how to use the SMART format for an inspiring graphic designer;

- **Specific**: Narrow down your goal and make it as clear and precise as possible. For example, instead of saying, "I want to draw," an inspiring graphic designer could set a specific goal like, "I want to become proficient in graphic design, build a professional portfolio, and work for a design agency."

- **Measurable**: You want to be able to measure your goal so you can track progress and stay motivated. For example, "I will spend the next six months studying graphic design using popular design software like Adobe Photoshop and Illustrator, then build at least ten unique projects for my portfolio."

- **Achievable**: To make the goal achievable, you could say, "I will enroll in an online graphic design course for beginners and join online communities for graphic designers to get feedback on my work."

- **Relevant**: Relevant goals are worthwhile, align with other things in your life, and are the right time to do them. For example, "Since I enjoy drawing and am interested in digital media, mastering graphic design will help me pursue a career that aligns with my interests."

- **Time-bound:** Finally, SMART goals should have a deadline so you stay on track. When do you plan on achieving your goal? For example, "I will complete all the required coursework to be proficient in graphic design, build a portfolio, and apply for entry-level design jobs within ten months of starting the course."

Sometimes it's better to break up your goals into short and long-term goals. What can get done right away? What's going to take more time to achieve? For example, say you want to start teaching yoga. Short-term goals could include getting certified in teaching yoga, creating promotional materials advertising on social media, and securing a teaching venue. Long-term goals could be opening your own yoga studio and organizing yoga retreats worldwide.

You'll need to consider potential challenges and solutions to get started. Say you're having difficulty attracting students to your class. One solution would be to offer the first class for free or collaborate with businesses in the local wellness community for mutual promotions.

Develop a plan to help you navigate the path efficiently. You might need to research, learn new skills, or make pivotal career decisions. For example, your yoga plan could include a vision statement, goals, action steps, specific tasks to follow, a way to track your progress, potential challenges and solutions, and a way to review your plan periodically. This will help you stay on track.

PURSUE

Start where you're at and take it one step at a time. There's no need to rush through this part.

FIND A MENTOR

The purpose of a mentor is to help you see the potential in yourself that you cannot see yourself.

~ Oprah Winfrey

Having a mentor can mean the difference between early success and taking a lifetime to achieve your goals. Mentors are experts in their field and have been around long enough to see it all. You get to learn from their mistakes, what worked for them and what didn't, and use their wisdom as a guide.

Mentors help mentees stay on track and refine their path as needed. They help you develop your skills through feedback and instruction, can introduce you to their network and job opportunities, and can increase your confidence and help you grow into the person you want to become.

Using the yoga example, you could seek out successful yoga teachers and studio owners to mentor you. You could also introduce yourself to the local health food shops, acupuncture clinics, pilates studios, gyms, and other professions in the health community who have successful businesses. Once you find one you want to work with, reach out to them and let them know why you admire their work and what kind of guidance you're seeking. This is where being clear in your goals will come in handy.

When looking for a mentor ask yourself these questions;

- What are my goals?
- What qualities am I looking for in a mentor?
- What kind of feedback am I looking for?
- What can I offer in return?
- Am I ready for constructive criticism?
- Do I want this to be in person or online?

The value of a mentor is priceless when it comes to achieving personal growth and success. They open doors to new opportunities, offer invaluable insight, and help transform your aspirations into reality. If you're serious about growth, then don't skip this step.

FOLLOW YOUR CURIOSITY

Finally, be willing and daring enough to follow your curiosity. There are enough people in this world to do the work you're not interested in, so be brave and go after what inspires you. The path may take you someplace better than you expected.

When pursuing your goals, start with bite-size pieces and build momentum over time. There's no need to take on big pursuits in the beginning. Find your Ikigai, take action, find a mentor, and remember that no matter how small, focus on one thing at a time. This sets you up for little wins and motivates you to continue moving forward.

Bring it all together.

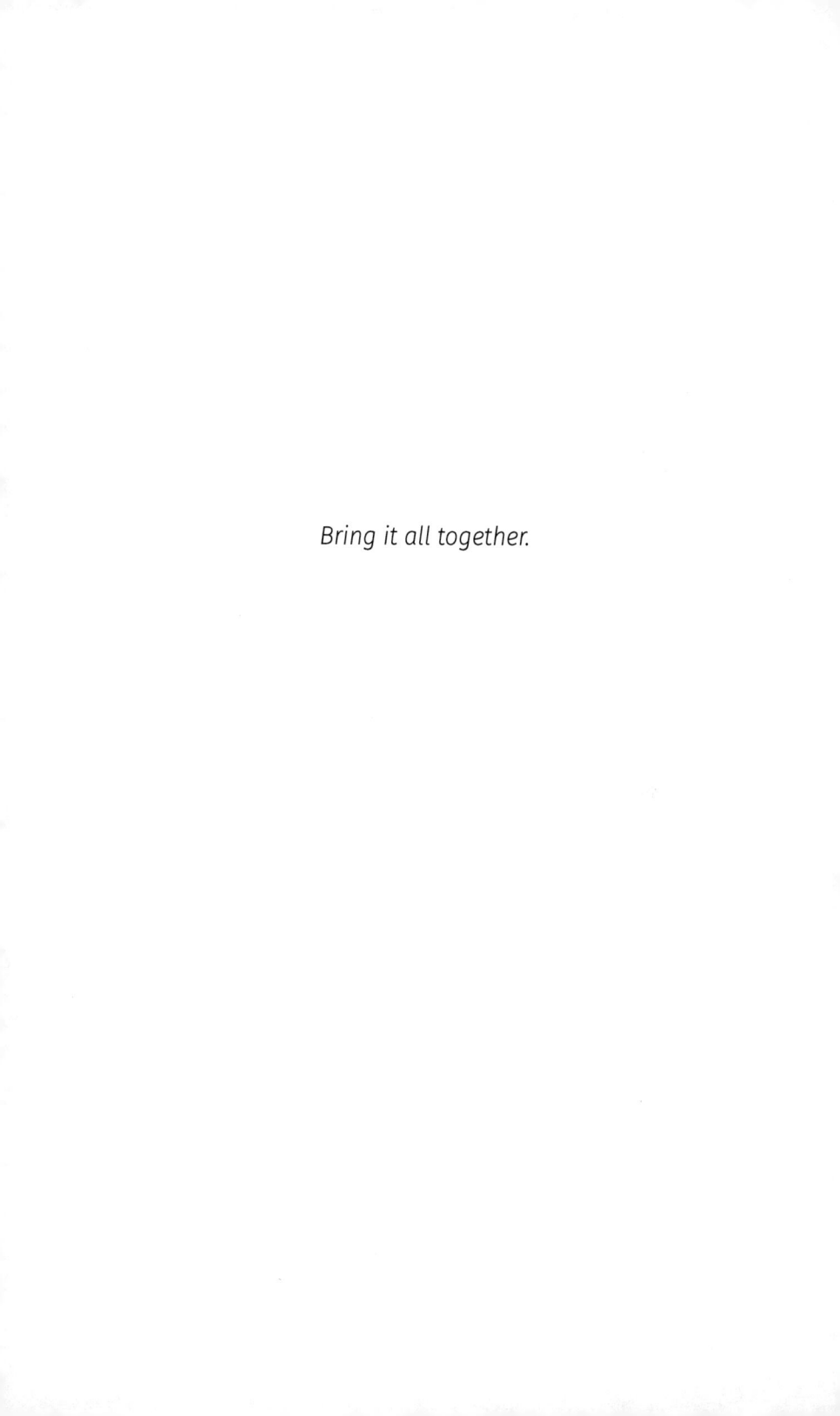

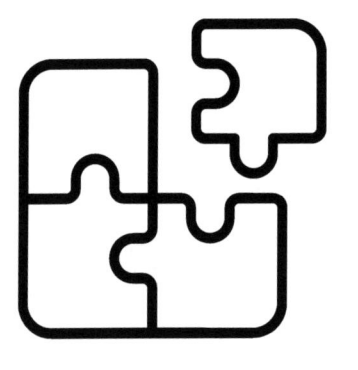

Integrate

*A person with outward courage dares to die;
a person with inward courage dares to live.*

~ Lao Tzu

Congratulations on making it to the end of this book. Now it's time for you to put everything you learned into action. My intention for writing this book was to help you learn the foundations of lifelong health and happiness so there's less chance of toppling over when life gets unpredictable. No matter what brought you here, you have the power to improve your life. From changing your mindset, to understanding the impacts of diet, exercise, sleep and stress, to cultivating better relationships and finding your higher purpose—you are in charge of your life and well-being.

While you may not be where you want to be today, with time and effort, you can create the life you want. The key is to go at your own pace, never stop learning, and never stop improving. Here's a recap of everything we went over;

REWIRE

- Use the power of your mind to do difficult things and change your life.
- Believe in yourself and be willing to push through the discomfort that the unknown brings.
- Become aware of the negative scrips running in your mind, challenge them, and rewrite them so you can have a better life.
- Use mental imagery to create your future.
- Let go of self-defeating habits by reinventing yourself and changing your identity.
- Focus on the good in your life, be grateful for al that you have, and practice self-love.
- Unclutter your mind and use meditation to pause the stories in your head.

EAT

- What we eat plays a direct role in how we look, think, feel, and act.
- Focusing on nutrient-dense foods is the key to better health.
- Avoid ultra-processed foods like chips, soda, donuts, candy, and margarine.

INTEGRATE

- Eat minimally processed foods like yogurt, frozen fruit and veggies, canned tomato sauce, and cold pressed oils.

- Eat mostly real food like unprocessed fruits, veggies, whole grains, and animal products.

- Eat primarily plants, but animal products from healthy animals are okay.

- Be 'vegicurious' and feed your microbiome with as many plant fibers as possible.

- Eat healthy fats like avocados, nuts, seeds, eggs and fatty fish and avoid refined seed and vegetable oils and hydrogenated fats.

- Don't burn your fat. Keep it below it's smoking point to avoid harmful chemicals.

- Eat every color of the rainbow to get a wide array of nutrients.

- Stay hydrated and drink half your weight in ounces daily.

- Be mindful of your portion sizes and don't overeat.

- Space your meals four hours apart and shrink your eating window down to 12 hours or less.

- Choose healthier cooking methods. Steaming, dehydrating, slow cooking, and boiling are healthier than grilling, microwaving, or deep frying.

- Eat organic whenever possible and avoid foods sprayed with pesticides.

BEING WELL

- Buy antibiotic and hormone free animal products.
- Prep your meals ahead of time to avoid overeating on ultra-processed foods.
- Keep the majority of your meals simple and don't overcomplicate it.
- Eat slowly, savor each bite, and enjoy your food!

MOVE

- Beyond physical health, movement plays a role in our mood, how we think, how well we sleep, and overall well-being.
- Start where you're at and don't over do it. Build your confidence, strength, and endurance overtime.
- Aim for 150 of moderate aerobic or 75 minutes of vigorous activity weekly.
- The best kind of exercise is whatever you like and are willing to do repeatedly.
- Walking, jogging, running, cycling, swimming, resistance bands, yoga, and racket sports are all great ways to move the body.
- Overcome exercise anxiety by going at your own pace.
- Bring a friend along and workout together.

INTEGRATE

SLEEP

- Quality sleep is as important as good nutrition and exercise. It's the reset button for the mind, body, and spirit.

- Learn about the sleep-wake cycle and stages of sleep.

- Sleep better by building good habits one at a time.

- Get 5 - 10 minutes of early morning sunlight.

- Limit caffeine intake or don't indulge at all.

- Avoid alcohol. If you must indulge, limit to one drink, hydrate, and stop early.

- Stop eating three hours before bedtime. Your dinner should consist of foods that encourage a good night's rest.

- Move your body during the day, but don't exercise three hours before bedtime to avoid overstimulation.

- Create sleep rituals like taking a warm bath, turning on soft music, or breathing exercises.

- Keep your bedroom clean, comfortable, and cool.

- Shut off all screens an hour before bed. Listening to soft music, an audiobook, or podcast is fine.

- Get heavy topics off your chest before laying down to sleep.

- Once you're sleeping well, create a sleep schedule and stick to it.

BEING WELL

- Get out of bed if you can't sleep—meditate, journal, or read a calming book.
- Make love and climax to help with falling asleep.
- Keep your naps less than 20 minutes and no later than 3:00 pm.
- If you can't sleep, try natural and non-habit forming sleep remedies.

RELAX

- Stress is linked to many chronic diseases and mitigating it is paramount for maintaining balance in life.
- Humans aren't built for chronic stress.
- Figure out what your triggers are and how to avoid them.
- Know how stress affects and manifests in your body.
- Exercise to burn off stress and lower stress hormones.
- Relax harder. Try deep breathing exercises and progressive muscle relaxation.
- Spend time out in nature to reset your nervous systems.
- Journal and write out your feelings.
- Eat foods that combat stress such as complex carbohydrates, fatty fish, berries, bananas, citrus, and poultry.

INTEGRATE

- Instead of alcohol, sugar, or caffeine to cope with stress, choose healthier vices such as herbal teas, adaptogens, green smoothies, and decaf coffee.
- Find ways to laugh and play.
- Get good quality and quantity sleep so you can handle stress better.
- Lean on friends to help you through difficult times.
- Unplug and monitor how much negativity you consume on social media and the news.
- Get good at managing your time.
- Learn to say no when needed.

DETOX

- Support your body's natural detoxification system by avoiding toxins, eating nutritious foods, exercising, and getting quality sleep.
- Stop putting toxins in your body.
- Replace toxic cleaning, household, and personal care products with green, unscented and chemical free ones.
- Drink plenty of water to flush out your system.
- Focus on foods that support liver biotransformation and open the detox pathways.
- Eat a fiber rich diet to help with elimination.

BEING WELL

- Eat organic whenever possible and avoid foods heavily sprayed with pesticides as the liver has to break them down.

- Give your gut a break. An overnight fast of 12 or more hours supports your detoxification organs and pathways.

- Consider supplements that support the liver and detoxification pathways.

- Avoid substances that burden the liver.

- Exercise regularly to move the lymphatic system.

- Prioritize sleep so the brain and central nervous system can remove waste products.

- Find ways to relax as stress hormones interfere with detoxification.

- Dry brush your body to stimulate the lymphatic system and drainage.

- Get a massage to encourage lymphatic drainage.

- Sit in a traditional or infrared sauna to support detoxification.

- Take an epsom salt bath.

- Use an air purifier to clean the air in your home an office.

- Invest in a water filtration system that specifically filters out the contaminants in your area.

INTEGRATE

CONNECT

- Community is the foundation upon which we build our lives.

- The health of your relationships are markers of overall well-being.

- Work on yourself first. Know who you are and what you want.

- Water your relationships with the 5As—affection, appreciation, attention, acceptance, availability.

- Notice what you like about people more than what you don't.

- Make new friends throughout your lifetime. New friendships help you grow.

- Pick your battles and don't fight over small things.

- Reevaluate the top 5 people you spend the most time with.

- Influence your friends to be and do better.

- Limit the time spent with negative people and let go of people who don't bring out the best in you.

- Stay connected through in person meet ups, talking on the phone, text, or internet.

PURSUE

- A life led by purpose, values, and goals is the foundation of lifelong health and happiness.
- Use the Ikigai formula to find your purpose.
- Figure out what you love doing.
- Figure out what the world needs in relation to what you love doing.
- Figure out what you are good at and how you can contribute to the world.
- Figure out what you can get paid for with what you love doing, what the world needs, and what you are good at.
- Take action by using the SMART format and a systems approach.
- Find a mentor who can speed up the process and hold you accountable.
- Follow your curiosity.

FINAL THOUGHTS

While some may view the above elements as separate entities, they are deeply intertwined. They have a bidirectional relationship, meaning when one is out of balance, so are the others. Physically healthy individuals tend to be happier and more fulfilled, while those struggling with their health tend to be less happy. By nurturing one area you can no doubt elevate

INTEGRATE

all. However, if you truly want to change your life, you must actively work on improving all areas of well-being. Change is an ever unfolding lifelong journey. Staying on the path to a healthier, happier you takes courage and commitment to your own growth. While it may seem daunting at first, every decision is an opportunity to shape your well-being. Celebrate every twist and turn, as they too are your teachers. Build yourself a strong foundation in health and happiness and witness your life transform.

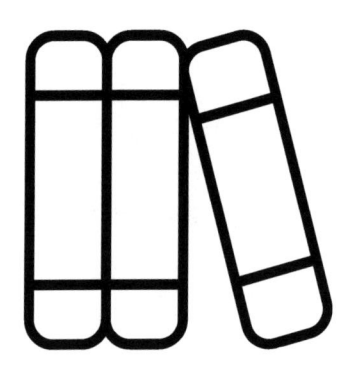

Resources

Scan the QR code below to access free guided meditations, self-discovery worksheets, and additional resources for this book. These resources are my gift to you to help deepen your understanding of yourself, and create a more immersive experience on your journey to Being Well.

References

INTRO

1. Farhud D. D. (2015). Impact of Lifestyle on Health. Iranian journal of public health, 44(11), 1442–1444.

2. About Chronic Disease | CDC. Retrieved on 12/2/2023. **https://www.cdc.gov/chronicdisease/about/index.htm**

REWIRE

1. Seitza, R., Angel, H. (2020). Belief formation – A driving force for brain evolution. Brain and Cognition. **https://www.sciencedirect.com/science/article/pii/S0278262619303860**

2. Kumar, A., Pareek, V., Faiq, M. A., Ghosh, S. K., & Kumari, C. (2019). ADULT NEUROGENESIS IN HUMANS: A Review of Basic Concepts, History, Current Research, and Clinical Implications. Innovations in clinical neuroscience, 16(5-6), 30–37. https://www.ncbi.nlm.nih.gov/pmc/articles/PMC6659986/

3. Alana L Conner, Danielle Z Boles, Hazel Rose Markus, Jennifer L Eberhardt, Alia J Crum, Americans' Health Mindsets: Content, Cultural Patterning, and Associations With Physical and Mental Health, Annals of Behavioral Medicine, Volume 53, Issue 4, April 2019, Pages 321–332, **https://doi.org/10.1093/abm/kay041**

4. Renner, F., Murphy, F. C., Ji, J. L., Manly, T., & Holmes, E. A. (2019). Mental imagery as a "motivational amplifier" to promote activities. Behaviour research and therapy, 114, 51–59. **https://doi.org/10.1016/j.brat.2019.02.002**

5. Reddan, M., Wager, T. (2018). Attenuating Neural threat expression with imagination. Cell Press. **https://www.cell.com/neuron/fulltext/S0896-6273(18)30955-3?_returnURL=https%3A%2F%2Flinkinghub.elsevier.com%2Fretrieve%2Fpii%2FS0896627318309553%3Fshowall%3Dtrue**

6. Pearson, J. The human imagination: the cognitive neuroscience of visual mental imagery. Nat Rev Neurosci 20, 624–634 (2019). **https://doi.org/10.1038/s41583-019-0202-9**

7. Pearson, J., Naselaris, T., Holmes, E. A., & Kosslyn, S. M. (2015). Mental Imagery: Functional Mechanisms and Clinical Applications. Trends in cognitive sciences, 19(10), 590–602. **https://doi.org/10.1016/j.tics.2015.08.003**

8. Budnik-Przybylska, D., Syty, P., Kaźmierczak, M. et al. Exploring the influence of personal factors on physiological responses to mental imagery in sport. Sci Rep 13, 2628 (2023) **https://doi.org/10.1038/s41598-023-29811-6**

9. Rhodes, J., Nedza, K., May, J., Jenkins, T. & Stone, T. (2021). From couch to ultra marathon: using functional imagery training to enhance motivation. Journal of Imagery Research in Sport and Physical Activity, 16(1), 20210011. https://doi.org/10.1515/jirspa-2021-0011

10. Lede, E., Meleady, R., Sager, C. (2019). Optimizing the influence of social norms interventions: Applying social identity insights to motivate residential water conservation. Journal of Applied Psychology. **https://doi.org/10.1016/j.jenvp.2019.02.011**

11. Vaish, A., Grossmann, T., & Woodward, A. (2008). Not all emotions are created equal: the negativity bias in social-emotional development. Psychological bulletin, 134(3), 383–403. **https://doi.org/10.1037/0033-2909.134.3.383**

12. Müller-Pinzler, L., Czekalla, N., Mayer, A.V. et al. Negativity-bias in forming beliefs about own abilities. Sci Rep 9, 14416 (2019). **https://doi.org/10.1038/s41598-019-50821-w**

REFERENCES

13. Newman, D. B., Gordon, A. M., & Mendes, W. B. (2021). Comparing daily physiological and psychological benefits of gratitude and optimism using a digital platform. Emotion (Washington, D.C.), 21(7), 1357–1365. **https://doi.org/10.1037/emo0001025**

14. Shokrpour, N., Sheidaie, S., Amirkhani, M., Bazrafkan, L., & Modreki, A. (2021). Effect of positive thinking training on stress, anxiety, depression, and quality of life among hemodialysis patients: A randomized controlled clinical trial. Journal of education and health promotion, 10, 225. **https://doi.org/10.4103/jehp.jehp_1120_20**

15. Stephen M. Yoshimura & Kassandra Berzins (2017) Grateful experiences and expressions: the role of gratitude expressions in the link between gratitude experiences and well-being, Review of Communication, 17:2, 106-118, DOI: **10.1080/15358593.2017.1293836**

16. Mills, P. J., Redwine, L., Wilson, K., Pung, M. A., Chinh, K., Greenberg, B. H., Lunde, O., Maisel, A., Raisinghani, A., Wood, A., & Chopra, D. (2015). The role of gratitude in spiritual well-being in asymptomatic heart failure patients. Spirituality in Clinical Practice, 2(1), 5–17. **https://doi.org/10.1037/scp0000050**

17. Nawa, N.E., Yamagishi, N. Enhanced academic motivation in university students following a 2-week online gratitude journal intervention. BMC Psychol 9, 71 (2021). **https://doi.org/10.1186/s40359-021-00559-w**

18. Tani Y, Koyama Y, Doi S, Sugihara G, Machida M, Amagasa S, Murayama H, Inoue S, Fujiwara T, Shobugawa Y. Association between gratitude, the brain and cognitive function in older adults: Results from the NEIGE study. Arch Gerontol Geriatr. 2022 May-Jun;100:104645. doi: 10.1016/j.archger.2022.104645. Epub 2022 Jan 30. PMID: 35123174.

19. Burgstahler MS, Stenson MC. Effects of guided mindfulness meditation on anxiety and stress in a pre-healthcare college student population: a pilot study. J Am Coll Health. 2020 Aug-Sep;68(6):666-672. doi: 10.1080/07448481.2019.1590371. Epub 2019 Apr 2. PMID: 30939081.

20. Basso, J. C., McHale, A., Ende, V., Oberlin, D. J., & Suzuki, W. A. (2019). Brief, daily meditation enhances attention, memory, mood, and emotional regulation in non-experienced meditators. Behavioural brain research, 356, 208–220. **https://doi.org/10.1016/j.bbr.2018.08.023**

21. Parmentier, F. B. R., García-Toro, M., García-Campayo, J., Yañez, A. M., Andrés, P., & Gili, M. (2019). Mindfulness and Symptoms of Depression and Anxiety in the General Population: The Mediating Roles of Worry, Rumination, Reappraisal and Suppression. Frontiers in psychology, 10, 506. **https://doi.org/10.3389/fpsyg.2019.00506**

EAT

1. Chen, Y., Michalak, M., & Agellon, L. B. (2018). Importance of Nutrients and Nutrient Metabolism on Human Health. The Yale journal of biology and medicine, 91(2), 95–103.

2. Center for Disease Control and PRevention (CDC). Poor Nutrition. Retrieved on 12/2/23. **https://www.cdc.gov/chronicdisease/resources/publications/factsheets/nutrition.htm#:~:text=Consuming%20unhealthy%20food%20and%20beverages,in%20postmenopausal%20women,%20and%20colorectal**

3. Nemec K. (2020). Cultural Awareness of Eating Patterns in the Health Care Setting. Clinical liver disease, 16(5), 204–207. **https://doi.org/10.1002/cld.1019**

4. Gramza-Michałowska A. (2020). The Effects of Ultra-Processed Food Consumption-Is There Any Action Needed?. Nutrients, 12(9), 2556. **https://doi.org/10.3390/nu12092556**

5. Martínez Leo EE, Segura Campos MR. Effect of ultra-processed diet on gut microbiota and thus its role in neurodegenerative diseases. Nutrition. 2020 Mar;71:110609. doi: 10.1016/j.nut.2019.110609. Epub 2019 Oct 11. PMID: 31837645.

6. Hall, K., Ayuketah, A., Brychta, R., Cao, H., Cassimatis, T., Chen, C., et al. (2019). Ultra-processed diets cause excess calorie intake and weight gain.: An inpatient randomized controlled trial of ad libitum food intake. Cell Metabolism. **https://doi.org/10.1016/j.cmet.2019.05.008**

REFERENCES

7. Jardim MZ, Costa BVL, Pessoa MC, Duarte CK. Ultra-processed foods increase noncommunicable chronic disease risk. Nutr Res. 2021 Nov;95:19-34. doi: 10.1016/j.nutres.2021.08.006. Epub 2021 Sep 11. PMID:34798466.

8. Bansal, S., Connolly, M., & Harder, T. (2021). Impact of a Whole-Foods, Plant-Based Nutrition Intervention on Patients Living with Chronic Disease in an Underserved Community. American journal of lifestyle medicine, 16(3), 382–389. **https://doi.org/ 10.1177/15598276211018159**

9. Subramaniam S, Selvaduray KR, Radhakrishnan AK. Bioactive Compounds: Natural Defense Against Cancer? Biomolecules. 2019 Nov 21;9(12):758. doi: 10.3390/biom9120758. PMID: 31766399; PMCID: PMC6995630

10. McMacken, M., & Shah, S. (2017). A plant-based diet for the prevention and treatment of type 2 diabetes. Journal of geriatric cardiology : JGC, 14(5), 342–354. **https://doi.org/10.11909/ j.issn.1671-5411.2017.05.009**

11. Davis, H., Magistrali, A., Butler, G., & Stergiadis, S. (2022). Nutritional Benefits from Fatty Acids in Organic and Grass-Fed Beef. Foods (Basel, Switzerland), 11(5), 646. **https://doi.org/ 10.3390/foods11050646**

12. Fu, J., Zheng, Y., Gao, Y., & Xu, W. (2022). Dietary Fiber Intake and Gut Microbiota in Human Health. Microorganisms, 10(12), 2507. **https://doi.org/10.3390/microorganisms10122507**

13. McDonald, D., Hyde, E., Debelius, J. W., Morton, J. T., Gonzalez, A., Ackermann, G., Aksenov, A. A., Behsaz, B., Brennan, C., Chen, Y., DeRight Goldasich, L., Dorrestein, P. C., Dunn, R. R., Fahimipour, A. K., Gaffney, J., Gilbert, J. A., Gogul, G., Green, J. L., Hugenholtz, P., Humphrey, G., … Knight, R. (2018). American Gut: an Open Platform for Citizen Science Microbiome Research. mSystems, 3(3), e00031-18. **https://doi.org/10.1128/ mSystems.00031-18**

14. Center for Disease Control and Prevention. Americans Slightly Taller, Munich Heavier Than Four Decades Ago. Retrieved on 12/2/23. **https://www.cdc.gov/nchs/pressroom/04news/ americans.htm**

15. NCD Risk Factor Collaboration (NCD-RisC). Worldwide trends in diabetes since 1980: a pooled analysis of 751 population-based studies with 4.4 million participants. Lancet. 2016 Apr 9;387(10027):1513-1530. doi: 10.1016/S0140-6736(16)00618-8. Epub 2016 Apr 6. Erratum in: Lancet. 2017 Feb 4;389(10068):e2. PMID: 27061677; PMCID: PMC5081106.

16. Reddy P, Jialal I. Biochemistry, Fat Soluble Vitamins. [Updated 2022 Sep 19]. In: StatPearls [Internet]. Treasure Island (FL): StatPearls Publishing; 2023 Jan-. Available from: **https://www.ncbi.nlm.nih.gov/books/NBK534869/**

17. DiNicolantonio, J. J., & O'Keefe, J. H. (2017). Good Fats versus Bad Fats: A Comparison of Fatty Acids in the Promotion of Insulin Resistance, Inflammation, and Obesity. Missouri medicine, 114(4), 303–307.

18. DiNicolantonio, J. J., & O'Keefe, J. H. (2018). Omega-6 vegetable oils as a driver of coronary heart disease: the oxidized linoleic acid hypothesis. Open heart, 5(2), e000898. **https://doi.org/10.1136/openhrt-2018-000898**

19. Ganesan K, Sukalingam K, Xu B. Impact of consumption of repeatedly heated cooking oils on the incidence of various cancers-A critical review. Crit Rev Food Sci Nutr. 2019;59(3):488-505. doi: 10.1080/10408398.2017.1379470. Epub 2017 Oct 20. PMID: 28925728.

20. Baig, A., Zubair, M., Sumrra, S. H., Nazar, M. F., Zafar, M. N., Jabeen, K., Hassan, M. B., & Rashid, U. (2022). Heating effect on quality characteristics of mixed canola cooking oils. BMC chemistry, 16(1), 3. **https://doi.org/10.1186/s13065-022-00796-z**

21. Kummerow FA. The negative effects of hydrogenated trans fats and what to do about them. Atherosclerosis. 2009 Aug;205(2):458-65. doi: 10.1016/j.atherosclerosis.2009.03.009. Epub 2009 Mar 19. PMID:19345947.

22. Okamura, T., Hashimoto, Y., Majima, S., Senmaru, T., Ushigome, E., Nakanishi, N., Asano, M., Yamazaki, M., Takakuwa, H., Hamaguchi, M., & Fukui, M. (2021). Trans Fatty Acid Intake Induces Intestinal Inflammation and Impaired Glucose Tolerance. Frontiers in immunology, 12, 669672. **https://doi.org/10.3389/fimmu.2021.669672**

REFERENCES

23. Liu, Q., Wu, P., Zhou, P., & Luo, P. (2023). Levels and Health Risk Assessment of Polycyclic Aromatic Hydrocarbons in Vegetable Oils and Frying Oils by Using the Margin of Exposure (MOE) and the Incremental Lifetime Cancer Risk (ILCR) Approach in China. Foods (Basel, Switzerland), 12(4), 811. **https://doi.org/10.3390/foods12040811**

24. Monjotin, N., Amiot, M. J., Fleurentin, J., Morel, J. M., & Raynal, S. (2022). Clinical Evidence of the Benefits of Phytonutrients in Human Healthcare. Nutrients, 14(9), 1712. **https://doi.org/10.3390/nu14091712**

25. Miller, M.D., Steinmaus, C., Golub, M.S. et al. Potential impacts of synthetic food dyes on activity and attention in children: a review of the human and animal evidence. Environ Health 21, 45 (2022). **https://doi.org/10.1186/s12940-022-00849-9**

26. Qi Zhang, Alexander A. Chumanevich, Ivy Nguyen, Anastasiya A. Chumanevich, Nora Sartawi, Jake Hogan, Minou Khazan, Quinn Harris, Bryson Massey, Ioulia Chatzistamou, Phillip J. Buckhaults, Carolyn E. Banister, Michael Wirth, James R. Hebert, E. Angela Murphy, Lorne J. Hofseth. The synthetic food dye, Red 40, causes DNA damage, causes colonic inflammation, and impacts the microbiome in mice. **https://doi.org/10.1016/j.toxrep.2023.08.006**

27. Potential Neurobehavioral Effects of Synthetic Food Dyes in Children. Office of Environmental Health Hazard Assessment. Retrieved on 12/5/23 from **https://oehha.ca.gov/media/downloads/risk-assessment/report/healthefftsassess041621.pdf**

28. Kobylewski, S., & Jacobson, M. F. (2012). Toxicology of food dyes. International journal of occupational and environmental health, 18(3), 220–246. **https://doi.org/10.1179/1077352512Z.00000000034**

29. Popkin, B. M., D'Anci, K. E., & Rosenberg, I. H. (2010). Water, hydration, and health. Nutrition reviews, 68(8), 439–458. **https://doi.org/10.1111/j.1753-4887.2010.00304.x**

30. Lorenzo, I., Serra-Prat, M., & Yébenes, J. C. (2019). The Role of Water Homeostasis in Muscle Function and Frailty: A Review. Nutrients, 11(8), 1857. **https://doi.org/10.3390/nu11081857**

31. Thornton S. N. (2016). Increased Hydration Can Be Associated with Weight Loss. Frontiers in nutrition, 3, 18. **https://doi.org/10.3389/fnut.2016.00018**

32. Liska, D., Mah, E., Brisbois, T., Barrios, P. L., Baker, L. B., & Spriet, L. L. (2019). Narrative Review of Hydration and Selected Health Outcomes in the General Population. Nutrients, 11(1), 70. **https://doi.org/10.3390/nu11010070**

33. Paoli, A., Tinsley, G., Bianco, A., & Moro, T. (2019). The Influence of Meal Frequency and Timing on Health in Humans: The Role of Fasting. Nutrients, 11(4), 719. **https://doi.org/10.3390/nu11040719**

34. Deloose, E., Janssen, P., Depoortere, I., & Tack, J. (2012). The migrating motor complex: control mechanisms and its role in health and disease. Nature reviews. Gastroenterology & hepatology, 9(5), 271–285. **https://doi.org/10.1038/nrgastro.2012.57**

35. Sutton, E. F., Beyl, R., Early, K. S., Cefalu, W. T., Ravussin, E., & Peterson, C. M. (2018). Early Time-Restricted Feeding Improves Insulin Sensitivity, Blood Pressure, and Oxidative Stress Even without Weight Loss in Men with Prediabetes. Cell metabolism, 27(6), 1212–1221.e3. **https://doi.org/10.1016/j.cmet.2018.04.010**

36. Moro, T., Tinsley, G., Pacelli, F. Q., Marcolin, G., Bianco, A., & Paoli, A. (2021). Twelve Months of Time-restricted Eating and Resistance Training Improves Inflammatory Markers and Cardiometabolic Risk Factors. Medicine and science in sports and exercise, 53(12), 2577–2585. **https://doi.org/10.1249/MSS.0000000000002738**

37. Chung, N., Bin, Y. S., Cistulli, P. A., & Chow, C. M. (2020). Does the Proximity of Meals to Bedtime Influence the Sleep of Young Adults? A Cross-Sectional Survey of University Students. International journal of environmental research and public health, 17(8), 2677. **https://doi.org/10.3390/ijerph17082677**

38. Deng X, Huang H, Huang S, Yang M, Wu J, Ci Z, He Y, Wu Z, Han L, Zhang D. Insight into the incredible effects of microwave heating: Driving changes in the structure, properties and functions of macromolecular nutrients in novel food. Front Nutr. 2022 Oct 13;9:941527. doi: 10.3389/fnut.2022.941527. PMID: 36313079; PMCID: PMC9607893

REFERENCES

39. Hussain, K. A., Romanova, S., Okur, I., Zhang, D., Kuebler, J., Huang, X., Wang, B., Fernandez-Ballester, L., Lu, Y., Schubert, M., & Li, Y. (2023). Assessing the Release of Microplastics and Nanoplastics from Plastic Containers and Reusable Food Pouches: Implications for Human Health. Environmental science & technology, 57(26), 9782–9792. **https://doi.org/10.1021/acs.est.3c01942**

40. Sun, Y., Liu, B., Snetselaar, L. G., Robinson, J. G., Wallace, R. B., Peterson, L. L., & Bao, W. (2019). Association of fried food consumption with all cause, cardiovascular, and cancer mortality: prospective cohort study. BMJ (Clinical research ed.), 364, k5420. **https://doi.org/10.1136/bmj.k5420**

41. Kori, R. K., Singh, M. K., Jain, A. K., & Yadav, R. S. (2018). Neurochemical and Behavioral Dysfunctions in Pesticide Exposed Farm Workers: A Clinical Outcome. Indian journal of clinical biochemistry : IJCB, 33(4), 372–381. **https://doi.org/10.1007/s12291-018-0791-5**

42. Pedroso, T. M. A., Benvindo-Souza, M., de Araújo Nascimento, F., Woch, J., Dos Reis, F. G., & de Melo E Silva, D. (2022). Cancer and occupational exposure to pesticides: a bibliometric study of the past 10 years. Environmental science and pollution research international, 29(12), 17464– 17475. **https://doi.org/10.1007/s11356-021-17031-2**

43. Mnif, W., Hassine, A. I., Bouaziz, A., Bartegi, A., Thomas, O., & Roig, B. (2011). Effect of endocrine disruptor pesticides: a review. International journal of environmental research and public health, 8(6), 2265–2303. **https://doi.org/10.3390/ijerph8062265**

44. Lee, G. H., & Choi, K. C. (2020). Adverse effects of pesticides on the functions of immune system. Comparative biochemistry and physiology. Toxicology & pharmacology : CBP, 235, 108789. **https://doi.org/10.1016/j.cbpc.2020.108789**

45. Ventola C. L. (2015). The antibiotic resistance crisis: part 1: causes and threats. P & T : a peer-reviewed journal for formulary management, 40(4), 277–283.

46. Zou, Z., Liu, W., Huang, C., Sun, C., & Zhang, J. (2020). First-Year Antibiotics Exposure in Relation to Childhood Asthma, Allergies, and Airway Illnesses. International journal of environmental

research and public health, 17(16), 5700. **https://doi.org/10.3390/ ijerph17165700**

47. Malekinejad, H., & Rezabakhsh, A. (2015). Hormones in Dairy Foods and Their Impact on Public Health - A Narrative Review Article. Iranian journal of public health, 44(6), 742–758.

MOVE

1. Nystoriak, M. A., & Bhatnagar, A. (2018). Cardiovascular Effects and Benefits of Exercise. Frontiers in cardiovascular medicine, 5, 135. **https://doi.org/10.3389/fcvm.2018.00135**

2. Prior, P. L., & Suskin, N. (2018). Exercise for stroke prevention. Stroke and vascular neurology, 3(2), 59–68. **https://doi.org/10.1136/ svn-2018-000155**

3. McTiernan, A., Friedenreich, C. M., Katzmarzyk, P. T., Powell, K. E., Macko, R., Buchner, D., Pescatello, L. S., Bloodgood, B., Tennant, B., Vaux-Bjerke, A., George, S. M., Troiano, R. P., Piercy, K. L., & 2018 PHYSICAL ACTIVITY GUIDELINES ADVISORY COMMITTEE*(2019). Physical Activity in Cancer Prevention and Survival: A Systematic Review. Medicine and science in sports and exercise, 51(6), 1252–1261. **https://doi.org/10.1249/ MSS.0000000000001937**

4. Kirwan, J. P., Sacks, J., & Nieuwoudt, S. (2017). The essential role of exercise in the management of type 2 diabetes. Cleveland Clinic journal of medicine, 84(7 Suppl 1), S15–S21. **https://doi.org/ 10.3949/ccjm.84.s1.03**

5. Alpsoy Ş. (2020). Exercise and Hypertension. Advances in experimental medicine and biology, 1228, 153–167. https://doi.org/ 10.1007/978-981-15- 1792-1_10

6. Alvarez-Jimenez, L., Moreno-Cabañas, A., Ramirez-Jimenez, M., Morales-Palomo, F., Ortega, J. F., & Mora-Rodriguez, R. (2022). Effectiveness of statins vs. exercise on reducing postprandial hypertriglyceridemia in dyslipidemic population: A systematic review and network meta-analysis. Journal of sport and health science, 11(5), 567–577. **https://doi.org/10.1016/j.jshs.2021.07.006**

REFERENCES

7. Pojednic, R., D'Arpino, E., Halliday, I., & Bantham, A. (2022). The Benefits of Physical Activity for People with Obesity, Independent of Weight Loss: A Systematic Review. International journal of environmental research and public health, 19(9), 4981. **https:// doi.org/10.3390/ijerph19094981**

8. Mahalakshmi, B., Maurya, N., Lee, S. D., & Bharath Kumar, V. (2020). Possible Neuroprotective Mechanisms of Physical Exercise in Neurodegeneration. International journal of molecular sciences, 21(16), 5895. **https://doi.org/10.3390/ijms21165895**

9. Schuch, F. B., Vancampfort, D., Richards, J., Rosenbaum, S., Ward, P. B., & Stubbs, B. (2016). Exercise as a treatment for depression: A meta-analysis adjusting for publication bias. Journal of psychiatric research, 77, 42–51. **https://doi.org/10.1016/ j.jpsychires.2016.02.023**

10. Henriksson, M., Wall, A., Nyberg, J., Adiels, M., Lundin, K., Bergh, Y., Eggertsen, R., Danielsson, L., Kuhn, H. G., Westerlund, M., David Åberg, N., Waern, M., & Åberg, M. (2022). Effects of exercise on symptoms of anxiety in primary care patients: A randomized controlled trial. Journal of affective disorders, 297, 26–34. **https://doi.org/10.1016/j.jad.2021.10.006**

11. Dolezal, B. A., Neufeld, E. V., Boland, D. M., Martin, J. L., & Cooper, C. B. (2017). Interrelationship between Sleep and Exercise: A Systematic Review. Advances in preventive medicine, 2017, 1364387. **https://doi.org/10.1155/2017/1364387**

12. Ramos, C., Gibson, G. R., Walton, G. E., Magistro, D., Kinnear, W., & Hunter, K. (2022). Systematic Review of the Effects of Exercise and Physical Activity on the Gut Microbiome of Older Adults. Nutrients, 14(3), 674. **https://doi.org/10.3390/nu14030674**

13. Simpson, R. J., Kunz, H., Agha, N., & Graff, R. (2015). Exercise and the Regulation of Immune Functions. Progress in molecular biology and translational science, 135, 355–380. **https://doi.org/ 10.1016/bs.pmbts.2015.08.001**

14. Piercy, K. L., Troiano, R. P., Ballard, R. M., Carlson, S. A., Fulton, J. E., Galuska, D. A., George, S. M., & Olson, R. D. (2018). The Physical Activity Guidelines for Americans. JAMA, 320(19), 2020–2028. **https://doi.org/10.1001/jama.2018.14854**

15. Fu, T. C., Wang, C. H., Lin, P. S., Hsu, C. C., Cherng, W. J., Huang, S. C.,Liu, M. H., Chiang, C. L., & Wang, J. S. (2013). Aerobic interval training improves oxygen uptake efficiency by enhancing cerebral and muscular hemodynamics in patients with heart failure. International journal of cardiology, 167(1), 41–50. **https://doi.org/10.1016/j.ijcard.2011.11.086**

16. Fyfe, J. J., Hamilton, D. L., & Daly, R. M. (2022). Minimal-Dose Resistance Training for Improving Muscle Mass, Strength, and Function: A Narrative Review of Current Evidence and Practical Considerations. Sports medicine (Auckland, N.Z.), 52(3), 463–479. **https://doi.org/10.1007/s40279-021-01605-8**

17. Woodyard C. (2011). Exploring the therapeutic effects of yoga and its ability to increase quality of life. International journal of yoga, 4(2), 49–54. **https://doi.org/10.4103/0973-6131.85485**

18. Dunsky A. (2019). The Effect of Balance and Coordination Exercises on Quality of Life in Older Adults: A Mini-Review. Frontiers in aging neuroscience, 11, 318. **https://doi.org/10.3389/fnagi.2019.00318**

19. Lee, D. C., Brellenthin, A. G., Thompson, P. D., Sui, X., Lee, I. M., & Lavie, C. J. (2017). Running as a Key Lifestyle Medicine for Longevity. Progress in cardiovascular diseases, 60(1), 45–55. **https://doi.org/10.1016/j.pcad.2017.03.005**

20. Zhao, Y., Hu, F., Feng, Y., Yang, X., Li, Y., Guo, C., Li, Q., Tian, G., Qie, R., Han, M., Huang, S., Wu, X., Zhang, Y., Wu, Y., Liu, D., Zhang, D., Cheng, C., Zhang, M., Yang, Y., Shi, X., … Hu, D. (2021). Association of Cycling with Risk of All-Cause and Cardiovascular Disease Mortality: A Systematic Review and Dose-Response Meta-analysis of Prospective Cohort Studies. Sports medicine (Auckland, N.Z.), 51(7), 1439–1448. **https://doi.org/10.1007/s40279-021-01452-7**

21. Green, S., Sakuls, P., & Levitt, S. (2021). Cycling for health: Improving health and mitigating the climate crisis. Canadian family physician Medecin de famille canadien, 67(10), 739–742. **https://doi.org/10.46747/cfp.6710739**

22. Lee, B. A., & Oh, D. J. (2015). Effect of regular swimming exercise on the physical composition, strength, and blood lipid of middle-

REFERENCES

aged women.Journal of exercise rehabilitation, 11(5), 266–271. **https://doi.org/10.12965/jer.150242**

23. Wong, A., Kwak, Y. S., Scott, S. D., Pekas, E. J., Son, W. M., Kim, J. S., & Park, S. Y. (2018). The effects of swimming training on arterial function, muscular strength, and cardiorespiratory capacity in postmenopausal women with stage 2 hypertension. Menopause (New York, N.Y.), 26(6), 653–658. **https://doi.org/10.1097/GME.0000000000001288**

24. Lopes, J. S. S., Machado, A. F., Micheletti, J. K., de Almeida, A. C., Cavina, A. P., & Pastre, C. M. (2019). Effects of training with elastic resistance versus conventional resistance on muscular strength: A systematic review and meta-analysis. SAGE open medicine, 7, 2050312119831116. **https://doi.org/10.1177/2050312119831116**

25. Farinatti, P. T., Rubini, E. C., Silva, E. B., & Vanfraechem, J. H. (2014). Flexibility of the elderly after one-year practice of yoga and calisthenics. International journal of yoga therapy, 24, 71–77.

26. Lau, C., Yu, R., & Woo, J. (2015). Effects of a 12-Week Hatha Yoga Intervention on Cardiorespiratory Endurance, Muscular Strength and Endurance, and Flexibility in Hong Kong Chinese Adults: A Controlled Clinical Trial. Evidence-based complementary and alternative medicine : eCAM, 2015, 958727. **https://doi.org/10.1155/2015/958727**

27. Cramer H. (2016). The Efficacy and Safety of Yoga in Managing Hypertension. Experimental and clinical endocrinology & diabetes :official journal, German Society of Endocrinology [and] German Diabetes Association, 124(2), 65–70. **https://doi.org/10.1055/s-0035-1565062**

28. Shree Ganesh, H. R., Subramanya, P., Rao M, R., & Udupa, V. (2021). Role of yoga therapy in improving digestive health and quality of sleep in an elderly population: A randomized controlled trial. Journal of bodywork and movement therapies, 27, 692–697. **https://doi.org/10.1016/j.jbmt.2021.04.012**

29. Estevao C. (2022). The role of yoga in inflammatory markers. Brain, behavior, & immunity - health, 20, 100421. **https://doi.org/10.1016/j.bbih.2022.100421**

30. Schnohr, P., O'Keefe, J. H., Holtermann, A., Lavie, C. J., Lange, P., Jensen, G. B., & Marott, J. L. (2018). Various Leisure-Time Physical Activities Associated With Widely Divergent Life Expectancies: The Copenhagen City Heart Study. Mayo Clinic proceedings, 93(12), 1775–1785. **https://doi.org/10.1016/j.mayocp.2018.06.025**

31. Oja, P., Kelly, P., Pedisic, Z., Titze, S., Bauman, A., Foster, C., Hamer, M., Hillsdon, M., & Stamatakis, E. (2017). Associations of specific types of sports and exercise with all-cause and cardiovascular-disease mortality: a cohort study of 80 306 British adults. British journal of sports medicine, 51(10), 812–817. **https://doi.org/10.1136/bjsports-2016-096822**

32. Chi, G., & Wang, L. (2022). The Association of Sports Participation With Depressive Symptoms and Anxiety Disorder in Adolescents. Frontiers in public health, 10, 860994. **https://doi.org/10.3389/fpubh.2022.860994**

SLEEP

1. Wilson, D., Driller, M., Winwood, P., Clissold, T., Johnston, B., & Gill, N. (2022). The Effectiveness of a Combined Healthy Eating, Physical Activity, and Sleep Hygiene Lifestyle Intervention on Health and Fitness of Overweight Airline Pilots: A Controlled Trial. Nutrients, 14(9), 1988. **https://doi.org/10.3390/nu14091988**

2. Besedovsky, L., Lange, T., & Haack, M. (2019). The Sleep-Immune Crosstalk in Health and Disease. Physiological reviews, 99(3), 1325–1380. **https://doi.org/10.1152/physrev.00010.2018**

3. Papatriantafyllou, E., Efthymiou, D., Zoumbaneas, E., Popescu, C. A., & Vassilopoulou, E. (2022). Sleep Deprivation: Effects on Weight Loss and Weight Loss Maintenance. Nutrients, 14(8), 1549. **https://doi.org/10.3390/nu14081549**

4. Jang, S. I., Lee, M., Han, J., Kim, J., Kim, A. R., An, J. S., Park, J. O., Kim, B. J., & Kim, E. (2020). A study of skin characteristics with long-term sleep restriction in Korean women in their 40s. Skin research and technology : official journal of International Society for Bioengineering and the Skin (ISBS) [and] International Society for Digital Imaging of Skin (ISDIS) [and] International Society for Skin Imaging (ISSI), 26(2), 193–199. **https://doi.org/10.1111/srt.12797**

REFERENCES

5. Copinschi, G., Leproult, R., & Spiegel, K. (2014). The important role of sleep in metabolism. Frontiers of hormone research, 42, 59–72. **https://doi.org/10.1159/000358858**

6. Kalmbach, D. A., Arnedt, J. T., Pillai, V., & Ciesla, J. A. (2015). The impact of sleep on female sexual response and behavior: a pilot study. The journal of sexual medicine, 12(5), 1221–1232. **https://doi.org/10.1111/jsm.12858**

7. Matenchuk, B. A., Mandhane, P. J., & Kozyrskyj, A. L. (2020). Sleep, circadian rhythm, and gut microbiota. Sleep medicine reviews, 53, 101340. **https://doi.org/10.1016/j.smrv.2020.101340**

8. Makarem, N., Shechter, A., Carnethon, M. R., Mullington, J. M., Hall, M. H., & Abdalla, M. (2019). Sleep Duration and Blood Pressure: Recent Advances and Future Directions. Current hypertension reports, 21(5), 33. **https://doi.org/10.1007/s11906-019-0938-7**

9. Klinzing, J. G., Niethard, N., & Born, J. (2019). Mechanisms of systems memory consolidation during sleep. Nature neuroscience, 22(10), 1598–1610. **https://doi.org/10.1038/s41593-019-0467-3**

10. Cox, R. C., & Olatunji, B. O. (2020). Sleep in the anxiety-related disorders: A meta-analysis of subjective and objective research. Sleep medicine reviews, 51, 101282. **https://doi.org/10.1016/j.smrv.2020.101282**

11. Dzierzewski, J. M., Donovan, E. K., Kay, D. B., Sannes, T. S., & Bradbrook, K. E. (2020). Sleep Inconsistency and Markers of Inflammation. Frontiers in neurology, 11, 1042. **https://doi.org/10.3389/fneur.2020.01042**

12. Mullington, J. M., Simpson, N. S., Meier-Ewert, H. K., & Haack, M. (2010). Sleep loss and inflammation. Best practice & research. Clinical endocrinology & metabolism, 24(5), 775–784. https://doi.org/10.1016/j.beem.2010.08.014

13. Sivertsen, B., Lallukka, T., Petrie, K. J., Steingrímsdóttir, Ó. A., Stubhaug, A., & Nielsen, C. S. (2015). Sleep and pain sensitivity in adults. Pain, 156(8), 1433–1439. **https://doi.org/10.1097/j.pain.0000000000000131**

14. Ramar, K., Malhotra, R. K., Carden, K. A., Martin, J. L., Abbasi-Feinberg, F., Aurora, R. N., Kapur, V. K., Olson, E. J., Rosen, C. L., Rowley, J. A., Shelgikar, A. V., & Trotti, L. M. (2021). Sleep is essential to health: an American Academy of Sleep Medicine position statement. Journal of clinical sleep medicine : JCSM : official publication of the American Academy of Sleep Medicine, 17(10), 2115–2119. **https://doi.org/10.5664/jcsm.9476**

15. Ramar, K., Malhotra, R. K., Carden, K. A., Martin, J. L., Abbasi-Feinberg, F., Aurora, R. N., Kapur, V. K., Olson, E. J., Rosen, C. L., Rowley, J. A., Shelgikar, A. V., & Trotti, L. M. (2021). Sleep is essential to health: an American Academy of Sleep Medicine position statement. Journal of clinical sleep medicine : JCSM : official publication of the American Academy of Sleep Medicine, 17(10), 2115–2119. **https://doi.org/10.5664/jcsm.9476**

16. Irwin M. R. (2015). Why sleep is important for health: a psychoneuroimmunology perspective. Annual review of psychology, 66, 143–172. **https://doi.org/10.1146/annurev-psych-010213-115205**

17. Patel AK, Reddy V, Shumway KR, et al. Physiology, Sleep Stages. [Updated 2022 Sep 7]. In: StatPearls [Internet]. Treasure Island (FL): StatPearls Publishing; 2023 Jan-. Available from: **https://www.ncbi.nlm.nih.gov/books/NBK526132/**

18. Reichert, C. F., Deboer, T., & Landolt, H. P. (2022). Adenosine, caffeine, and sleep-wake regulation: state of the science and perspectives. Journal of sleep research, 31(4), e13597. **https://doi.org/10.1111/jsr.13597**

19. Thakkar, M. M., Sharma, R., & Sahota, P. (2015). Alcohol disrupts sleep homeostasis. Alcohol (Fayetteville, N.Y.), 49(4), 299–310. **https://doi.org/10.1016/j.alcohol.2014.07.019**

20. He, S., Hasler, B. P., & Chakravorty, S. (2019). Alcohol and sleep-related problems. Current opinion in psychology, 30, 117–122. **https://doi.org/10.1016/j.copsyc.2019.03.007**

21. Uchida, S., Shioda, K., Morita, Y., Kubota, C., Ganeko, M., & Takeda, N. (2012). Exercise effects on sleep physiology. Frontiers in neurology, 3, 48. **https://doi.org/10.3389/fneur.2012.00048**

REFERENCES

22. Baniassadi, A., Manor, B., Yu, W., Travison, T., & Lipsitz, L. (2023). Nighttime ambient temperature and sleep in community-dwelling older adults. The Science of the total environment, 899, 165623. **https://doi.org/10.1016/j.scitotenv.2023.165623**

23. Baranwal, N., Yu, P. K., & Siegel, N. S. (2023). Sleep physiology, pathophysiology, and sleep hygiene. Progress in cardiovascular diseases, 77, 59–69. **https://doi.org/10.1016/j.pcad.2023.02.005**

24. Rusch, H. L., Rosario, M., Levison, L. M., Olivera, A., Livingston, W. S., Wu, T., & Gill, J. M. (2019). The effect of mindfulness meditation on sleep quality: a systematic review and meta-analysis of randomized controlled trials. Annals of the New York Academy of Sciences, 1445(1), 5–16. **https://doi.org/10.1111/nyas.13996**

25. Lastella, M., O'Mullan, C., Paterson, J. L., & Reynolds, A. C. (2019). Sex and Sleep: Perceptions of Sex as a Sleep Promoting Behavior in the General Adult Population. Frontiers in public health, 7, 33. **https://doi.org/10.3389/fpubh.2019.00033**

26. Yuan, C. S., Mehendale, S., Xiao, Y., Aung, H. H., Xie, J. T., & Ang-Lee, M. K. (2004). The gamma-aminobutyric acidergic effects of valerian and valerenic acid on rat brainstem neuronal activity. Anesthesia and analgesia, 98(2), 353–358. **https://doi.org/10.1213/01.ANE.0000096189.70405.A5**

27. Ngan, A., & Conduit, R. (2011). A double-blind, placebo-controlled investigation of the effects of Passiflora incarnata (passionflower) herbal tea on subjective sleep quality. Phytotherapy research : PTR, 25(8), 1153–1159. **https://doi.org/10.1002/ptr.3400**

28. Schwalfenberg, G. K., & Genuis, S. J. (2017). The Importance of Magnesium in Clinical Healthcare. Scientifica, 2017, 4179326. **https://doi.org/10.1155/2017/4179326**

29. Srivastava, J. K., Shankar, E., & Gupta, S. (2010). Chamomile: A herbal medicine of the past with bright future. Molecular medicine reports, 3(6), 895–901. https://doi.org/10.3892/mmr.2010.377

30. Yıldırım, D., Kocatepe, V., Can, G., Sulu, E., Akış, H., Şahin, G., & Aktay, E. (2020). The Effect of Lavender Oil on Sleep Quality and Vital Signs in Palliative Care: A Randomized Clinical Trial. Die Wirkung von Lavendelöl auf Schlafqualität und Vitalzeichen in der Palliativversorgung: Eine randomisierte klinische Studie.

Complementary medicine research, 27(5), 328–335. **https://doi.org/10.1159/000507319**

31. Rao, T. P., Ozeki, M., & Juneja, L. R. (2015). In Search of a Safe Natural Sleep Aid. Journal of the American College of Nutrition, 34(5), 436–447. **https://doi.org/10.1080/07315724.2014.926153**

RELAX

1. Liu, Y. Z., Wang, Y. X., & Jiang, C. L. (2017). Inflammation: The Common Pathway of Stress-Related Diseases. Frontiers in human neuroscience, 11, 316. **https://doi.org/10.3389/fnhum.2017.00316**

2. Mariotti A. (2015). The effects of chronic stress on health: new insights into the molecular mechanisms of brain-body communication. Future science OA, 1(3), FSO23. **https://doi.org/10.4155/fso.15.21**

3. Roberts, B. L., & Karatsoreos, I. N. (2021). Brain-body responses to chronic stress: a brief review. Faculty reviews, 10, 83. **https://doi.org/10.12703/r/10-83**

4. Nejade, R. M., Grace, D., & Bowman, L. R. (2022). What is the impact of nature on human health? A scoping review of the literature. Journal of global health, 12, 04099. **https://doi.org/10.7189/jogh.12.04099**

5. Jimenez, M. P., DeVille, N. V., Elliott, E. G., Schiff, J. E., Wilt, G. E., Hart, J. E., & James, P. (2021). Associations between Nature Exposure and Health: A Review of the Evidence. International journal of environmental research and public health, 18(9), 4790. **https://doi.org/10.3390/ijerph18094790**

6. Yap, Y., Slavish, D. C., Taylor, D. J., Bei, B., & Wiley, J. F. (2020). Bi-directional relations between stress and self-reported and actigraphy-assessed sleep: a daily intensive longitudinal study. Sleep, 43(3), zsz250. **https://doi.org/10.1093/sleep/zsz250**

DETOX

1. United Nations Environment Programme. (2020). An Assessment Report on Issues of Concern: Chemicals and Waste Issues Posing Risks to Human Health and the Environment. **https://**

REFERENCES

wedocs.unep.org/bitstream/handle/20.500.11822/33807/ARIC.pdf

2. Lamat H, Sauvant-Rochat MP, Tauveron I, et al. Metabolic syndrome and pesticides: a systematic review and meta-analysis. Environ Pollut. 2022;305:119288. doi:1016/j.envpol.2022.119288

3. Nicolopoulou-Stamati P, Maipas S, Kotampasi C, Stamatis P, Hens L. Chemical pesticides and human health: the urgent need for a new concept in agriculture. Front Public Health. 2016;4:148. doi:3389/fpubh.2016.00148

4. Sturm ET, Castro C, Mendez-Colmenares A, et al. Risk factors for brain health in agricultural work: a systematic review. Int J Environ Res Public Health. 2022;19(6):3373. doi:3390/ijerph19063373

5. Parida, L., & Patel, T. N. (2023). Systemic impact of heavy metals and their role in cancer development: a review. Environmental monitoring and assessment, 195(6), 766. https://doi.org/10.1007/s10661-023-11399-z

6. Bakulski, K. M., Seo, Y. A., Hickman, R. C., Brandt, D., Vadari, H. S., Hu, H., & Park, S. K. (2020). Heavy Metals Exposure and Alzheimer's Disease and Related Dementias. Journal of Alzheimer's disease : JAD, 76(4), 1215– 1242. https://doi.org/10.3233/JAD-200282

7. Rzymski, P., Tomczyk, K., Rzymski, P., Poniedziałek, B., Opala, T., & Wilczak, M. (2015). Impact of heavy metals on the female reproductive system. Annals of agricultural and environmental medicine : AAEM, 22(2), 259–264. https://doi.org/10.5604/12321966.1152077

8. Ma, Y., Liu, H., Wu, J., Yuan, L., Wang, Y., Du, X., Wang, R., Marwa, P. W., Petlulu, P., Chen, X., & Zhang, H. (2019). The adverse health effects of bisphenol A and related toxicity mechanisms. Environmental research, 176, 108575. https://doi.org/10.1016/j.envres.2019.108575

9. Persiani, E., Cecchettini, A., Ceccherini, E., Gisone, I., Morales, M. A., & Vozzi, F. (2023). Microplastics: A Matter of the Heart (and Vascular System). Biomedicines, 11(2), 264. https://doi.org/10.3390/biomedicines11020264

10. Chazelas, E., Pierre, F., Druesne-Pecollo, N., Esseddik, Y., Szabo de Edelenyi, F., Agaesse, C., De Sa, A., Lutchia, R., Gigandet, S., Srour, B., Debras, C., Huybrechts, I., Julia, C., Kesse-Guyot, E., Allès, B., Galan, P., Hercberg, S., Deschasaux-Tanguy, M., & Touvier, M. (2022). Nitrites and nitrates from food additives and natural sources and cancer risk: results from the NutriNet-Santé cohort. International journal of epidemiology, 51(4), 1106–1119. https://doi.org/10.1093/ije/dyac046

11. Trasande, L., Shaffer, R. M., Sathyanarayana, S., & COUNCIL ON ENVIRONMENTAL HEALTH (2018). Food Additives and Child Health. Pediatrics, 142(2), e20181410. https://doi.org/10.1542/peds.2018-1410

12. Mathur, K., Agrawal, R. K., Nagpure, S., & Deshpande, D. (2020). Effect of artificial sweeteners on insulin resistance among type-2 diabetes mellitus patients. Journal of family medicine and primary care, 9(1), 69–71. https://doi.org/10.4103/jfmpc.jfmpc_329_19

13. Debras, C., Chazelas, E., Sellem, L., Porcher, R., Druesne-Pecollo, N., Esseddik, Y., de Edelenyi, F. S., Agaësse, C., De Sa, A., Lutchia, R., Fezeu, L. K., Julia, C., Kesse-Guyot, E., Allès, B., Galan, P., Hercberg, S., Deschasaux-Tanguy, M., Huybrechts, I., Srour, B., & Touvier, M. (2022). Artificial sweeteners and risk of cardiovascular diseases: results from the prospective NutriNet-Santé cohort. BMJ (Clinical research ed.), 378, e071204. https://doi.org/10.1136/bmj-2022-071204

14. Shil, A., & Chichger, H. (2021). Artificial Sweeteners Negatively Regulate Pathogenic Characteristics of Two Model Gut Bacteria, E. coli and E. faecalis. International journal of molecular sciences, 22(10), 5228. https://doi.org/10.3390/ijms22105228

15. Yamashita, H., Matsuhara, H., Miotani, S., Sako, Y., Matsui, T., Tanaka, H., & Inagaki, N. (2017). Artificial sweeteners and mixture of food additives cause to break oral tolerance and induce food allergy in murine oral tolerance model for food allergy. Clinical and experimental allergy : journal of the British Society for Allergy and Clinical Immunology, 47(9), 1204–1213. https://doi.org/10.1111/cea.12928

16. Darbre, P. D. (2006). Environmental oestrogens, cosmetics and breast cancer. Best practice & research clinical endocrinology &

REFERENCES

metabolism, 20(1), 121-143. **https://doi.org/10.1016/ j.beem.2005.09.007**

17. Bilal, M., Mehmood, S., & Iqbal, H. M. (2020). The beast of beauty: environmental and health concerns of toxic components in cosmetics. Cosmetics, 7(1), 13. **https://doi.org/10.3390/ cosmetics7010013**

18. Ma, X., Nan, F., Liang, H., Shu, P., Fan, X., Song, X., Hou, Y., & Zhang, D. (2022). Excessive intake of sugar: An accomplice of inflammation. Frontiers in immunology, 13, 988481. **https:// doi.org/10.3389/fimmu.2022.988481**

19. Laguna, J. C., Alegret, M., Cofán, M., Sánchez-Tainta, A., Díaz-López, A., Martínez-González, M. A., Sorlí, J. V., Salas-Salvadó, J., Fitó, M., Alonso-Gómez, Á. M., Serra-Majem, L., Lapetra, J., Fiol, M., Gómez-Gracia, E., Pintó, X., Muñoz, M. A., Castañer, O., Ramírez-Sabio, J. B., Portu, J. J., Estruch, R., ... Ros, E. (2021). Simple sugar intake and cancer incidence, cancer mortality and all-cause mortality: A cohort study from the PREDIMED trial. Clinical nutrition (Edinburgh, Scotland), 40(10), 5269– 5277. **https:// doi.org/10.1016/j.clnu.2021.07.031**

20. Jacques, A., Chaaya, N., Beecher, K., Ali, S. A., Belmer, A., & Bartlett, S. (2019). The impact of sugar consumption on stress driven, emotional and addictive behaviors. Neuroscience and biobehavioral reviews, 103, 178– 199. **https://doi.org/10.1016/ j.neubiorev.2019.05.021**

21. Cao, C., Xiao, Z., Wu, Y., & Ge, C. (2020). Diet and Skin Aging-From the Perspective of Food Nutrition. Nutrients, 12(3), 870. **https://doi.org/10.3390/nu12030870**

22. Ambreen, G., Siddiq, A., & Hussain, K. (2020). Association of long-term consumption of repeatedly heated mix vegetable oils in different doses and hepatic toxicity through fat accumulation. Lipids in health and disease, 19(1), 69. **https://doi.org/10.1186/ s12944-020-01256-0**

23. Kalra A, Yetiskul E, Wehrle CJ, et al. Physiology, Liver. [Updated 2023 May 1]. In: StatPearls [Internet]. Treasure Island (FL): StatPearls Publishing; 2023 Jan-. Available from: **https:// www.ncbi.nlm.nih.gov/books/NBK535438/**

24. Jackson, E., Shoemaker, R., Larian, N., & Cassis, L. (2017). Adipose Tissue as a Site of Toxin Accumulation. Comprehensive Physiology, 7(4), 1085–1135. **https://doi.org/10.1002/cphy.c160038**

25. Pizzorno, J., & Pizzorno, L. (2021). Environmental Toxins Are a Major Cause of Bone Loss. Integrative medicine (Encinitas, Calif.), 20(1), 10–17.

26. Rodríguez, J., & Mandalunis, P. M. (2018). A Review of Metal Exposure and Its Effects on Bone Health. Journal of toxicology, 2018, 4854152. **https://doi.org/10.1155/2018/4854152**

27. Maurer, L. L., & Philbert, M. A. (2015). The mechanisms of neurotoxicity and the selective vulnerability of nervous system sites. Handbook of clinical neurology, 131, 61–70. **https://doi.org/10.1016/B978-0-444-62627-1.00005-6**

28. Liska, D., Mah, E., Brisbois, T., Barrios, P. L., Baker, L. B., & Spriet, L. L. (2019). Narrative Review of Hydration and Selected Health Outcomes in the General Population. Nutrients, 11(1), 70. **https://doi.org/10.3390/nu11010070**

29. Holscher H. D. (2017). Dietary fiber and prebiotics and the gastrointestinal microbiota. Gut microbes, 8(2), 172–184. **https://doi.org/10.1080/19490976.2017.1290756**

30. Sule, R. O., Condon, L., & Gomes, A. V. (2022). A Common Feature of Pesticides: Oxidative Stress-The Role of Oxidative Stress in Pesticide-Induced Toxicity. Oxidative medicine and cellular longevity, 2022, 5563759. **https://doi.org/10.1155/2022/5563759**

31. Crinnion W. J. (2010). Organic foods contain higher levels of certain nutrients, lower levels of pesticides, and may provide health benefits for the consumer. Alternative medicine review : a journal of clinical therapeutic, 15(1), 4–12.

32. Montgomery, D. R., Biklé, A., Archuleta, R., Brown, P., & Jordan, J. (2022). Soil health and nutrient density: preliminary comparison of regenerative and conventional farming. PeerJ, 10, e12848. **https://doi.org/10.7717/peerj.12848**

33. Zuvarox, T., & Belletieri, C. (2023). Malabsorption Syndromes. In StatPearls. StatPearls Publishing.

REFERENCES

34. Kumar, M., Ji, B., Babaei, P., Das, P., Lappa, D., Ramakrishnan, G., Fox, T. E., Haque, R., Petri, W. A., Bäckhed, F., & Nielsen, J. (2018). Gut microbiota dysbiosis is associated with malnutrition and reduced plasma amino acid levels: Lessons from genome-scale metabolic modeling. Metabolic engineering, 49, 128–142. **https://doi.org/10.1016/j.ymben.2018.07.018**

35. Buccellato, F. R., D'Anca, M., Serpente, M., Arighi, A., & Galimberti, D. (2022). The Role of Glymphatic System in Alzheimer's and Parkinson's Disease Pathogenesis. Biomedicines, 10(9), 2261. **https://doi.org/10.3390/biomedicines10092261**

CONNECT

1. Umberson, D. & Montez, J. (2010), Social relationships and health: a flashpoint for health policy. Journal of health and social behavior. **https://www.ncbi.nlm.nih.gov/pmc/articles/PMC3150158/** har

2. Christakis, N. A., & Fowler, J. H. (2007). The spread of obesity in a large social network over 32 years. The New England journal of medicine, 357(4), 370–379. **https://doi.org/10.1056/NEJMsa066082**

3. Harari, Y.N. (2015). Sapiens: A brief history of humankind.HarperCollins Publisher. **https://www.ynharari.com/book/sapiens-2/**

4. Marroquín, B., Vine, V., & Morgan, R. (2020). Mental health during the COVID-19 pandemic: Effects of stay-at-home policies, social distancing behavior, and social resources. Psychiatry research, 293, 113419. **https://doi.org/10.1016/j.psychres.2020.113419**

PURSUE

1. Willroth, E. C., Mroczek, D. K., & Hill, P. L. (2021). Maintaining sense of purpose in midlife predicts better physical health. Journal of psychosomatic research, 145, 110485. **https://doi.org/10.1016/j.jpsychores.2021.110485**

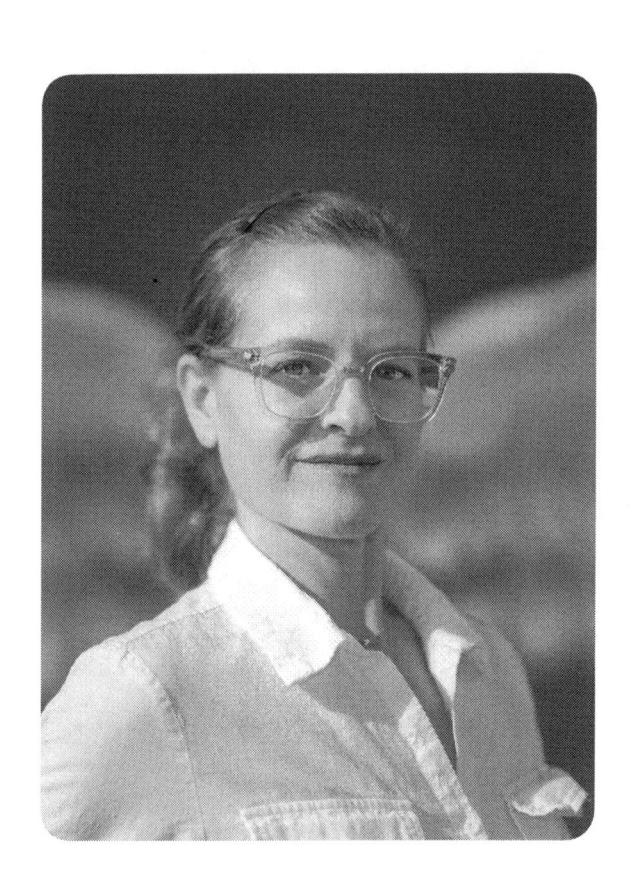

About the author

Dr. Ara's journey in the realm of wellness is as enriching as it is inspiring. With a master's degree from the Acupuncture and Integrative Medicine College in Berkeley, CA, her quest for knowledge took her across the world to Tianjin University in China, where she immersed herself in the ancient wisdom of Chinese Medicine.

Eager to share what she learned overseas, she opened a clinic in Southern California where she helped thousands of people regain their health through Eastern Medicine.

But her pursuit of comprehensive wellness solutions didn't stop there—she became a Functional Medicine practitioner, and later received a doctorate in Acupuncture & Chinese Medicine from the Pacific College of Health & Science.

All that to say, Dr. Ara's approach to wellness is a unique blend of time-honored practices and modern Functional Medicine. Her philosophy is simple—the path to wellness begins in the mind. It is not an end goal but a fascinating journey back to self.

What clients are saying

Dawna is wicked smart, a talented healer, and always knows what's going on with your body even if you don't. Dawna is humble, sweet, funny and always puts your health first. She's practical, honest and isn't adversed to integrating with Western Medicine if it truly works for you. She puts the individual first and never tries to indoctrinate you into her way of thinking or practicing.

~ Jess L

Dr. Ara is amazing. She is completely professional, and yet so warm and nurturing at the same time. I can tell that she really cares about her patients, and goes above and beyond the call of duty to take care of them.

~ Natalie T

BEING WELL

Dawna is an amazing healer. Its not just that she is attentive, a good listener, and has a soft touch, but she really knows what she is doing.

~ Jane M

Dawna has helped me with everything from garden variety stress to bizarre ailments that defy reason.

~ Anna S

I would recommend Dawna (and I have to friends) to anyone who is looking for an alternative approach to their situation/condition. Plus she's sweet, nice, and positive.

~ Barbara P

Dawna has changed my life and that hour I spend once a week with her I look forward to all week long.

~ Brenda M

Dawna is hands down one of the nicest practitioners you will ever meet. She truly cares about her patients and is an excellent listener.

~ Jennifer K

TESTIMONIALS

Dawna is not a normal acupuncturist. She is a HEALER who is passionate about what she does and you can tell in the ways she listens an treats your body.

~ Bora L

Dawna is absolutely great. So kind, and so talented. I have been going to her on and off for over a year, and every time I go I don't ever want to stop. Her services are amazing, and all my back problems have very much improved. I can't recommend her enough.

~ Nathalia F

Dawna is amazing. I totally love her. She is very attentive and is really committed to helping you address whatever problem/challenge you are having or simply to help you improve your overall health and well-being.

~ Raine J

I can not praise Dawna enough for her compassionate, intelligent, and tenacious approach. Dawna's holistic pedagogy helped me get through the remainder of my pregnancy with minimal stress and pain.

~ Alene T

BEING WELL

Excellent patient care. She listens to her patients and individualizes her treatment plans. Definitely recommend to others.

~ Liza S

I cannot say more wonderful things about Dawna. I've been seeing her for two months now for general health, stress, and fertility. I have not felt this great in a long time. My stress level is down, my mood is much better, and my cycles are regulated after years of being irregular. I would recommend Dawna to anyone who is looking to feel great both physically and mentally.

~ Kelley T

Dawna is a kind and calming person who treats her patients with care and like a friend. She takes the time to talk with her clients and answers all of their questions to best understand their needs.

~ CM H

Dawna is a great person to talk to and I look forward to our appointments. I have absolutely no reservation referring anyone to her, including my own parents who are now also patients of hers.

~ Melissa S

TESTIMONIALS

Dawna was comforting, understanding, listened to my concerns, and gave me much insight into what I'm feeling and why I'm feeling it without costing me an arm and a leg. Thank you Dawna.

~ Wesam N

She's extremely kind, interesting, reliable, and very willing to talk about how she's treating you, both in Chinese medicine terms and in more laymen terms. I highly recommend her!

~ Catherine A

Dawna Ara has given me my life back!

~ Pamela H

Dr. Ara is great. Super friendly and easy to talk to. I went to see her for chronic digestive issues and anxiety. I always felt so relaxed and calm afterwards.

~ Jesse F

Made in the USA
Columbia, SC
12 April 2024